AMERICAN MEDICAL ASSOCIATION
ESSENTIAL GUIDE TO
ASTHMA

Five percent of all adults and ten percent of all children living in the United States must cope with asthma, a serious, sometimes life-threatening chronic respiratory condition. The overall incidence of asthma is on the rise. The *American Medical Association Essential Guide to Asthma* provides a comprehensive yet readable overview of asthma as a disease, along with its diagnosis, prevention, and treatment.

Included in the book are thorough explanations of what happens in the body during an asthma attack and the wide array of substances in food, the environment, and in our own bodies that can trigger an attack. The book explains how asthma is diagnosed, which kinds of doctors treat asthma, and what other diseases sometimes mimic symptoms of asthma. Readers are given a wealth of specific instructions on what changes to make in their surroundings and their lifestyles in order to prevent asthma attacks. The chapter on treatments presents an up-to-date wrap-up of all medication and nonmedication treatments available.

The book explains how to create a detailed asthma emergency plan for times when regular treatments don't work. A number of lifestyle issues are addressed, including emotions, exercise, pregnancy, breast-feeding, and how to help children with asthma. Finally, the book is rounded out with a list of common asthma myths, a question-and-answer section, a list of asthma-related resources, and a glossary.

American
Medical
Association

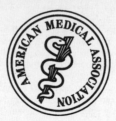

ESSENTIAL

GUIDE

TO

ASTHMA

POCKET BOOKS

New York   London   Toronto   Sydney   Tokyo   Singapore

An *Original* Publication of POCKET BOOKS

POCKET BOOKS, a division of Simon & Schuster Inc.
1230 Avenue of the Americas, New York, NY 10020

Library of Congress Cataloging-in-Publication Data

Essential guide to asthma / American Medical Association.
    p. cm.
    Includes bibliographical references and index.
    ISBN: 0-671-01013-1
    1. Asthma—Popular works.   I. American Medical Association.
RC591.E87   1998
616.2'38—dc21   98–15733
                                                CIP

First Pocket Books trade paperback printing August 1998

10 9 8 7 6 5 4 3 2

POCKET and colophon are registered trademarks of
Simon & Schuster Inc.

Cover design by Elizabeth Van Itallie
Cover photo by Tony Stone Images
Text design by Stanley S. Drate/Folio Graphics Co. Inc.

Printed in the U.S.A.

American Medical Association
Physicians dedicated to the health of America

Foreword

Millions of families deal with the realities of asthma every day. The good news is that with an appropriate treatment plan, people with asthma can now live full, productive lives; some have gone on to achieve great success in sports. The key to living a healthy life with asthma appears to be preventing emergencies; a comprehensive medical plan along with monitoring of the person's condition are the keys to stopping asthma attacks before they start. You and your family need accurate, clear, up-to-date information on asthma to help you manage it; that is why the American Medical Association decided to publish the *American Medical Association Essential Guide to Asthma*.

This book explains the main types of asthma medications and which ones might be recommended for people in different situations, for example, small children, people with other conditions such as heart problems, and so on. Using the information in this volume, you can work more effectively with your physician, or your child's physician, to treat asthma. You can also learn how to make modifications in your home environment that will help the person with asthma breathe easier.

The member physicians of the AMA offer you this information as part of a continuing effort to help you and your family stay healthy. If you have access to the Internet, look for more information about health and about physicians on the AMA website at **http://www.ama-assn.org**; if you need a physician, you can access information by specialty or by doctor's name under Physician Select: The Doctor Finder.

The American Medical Association wishes you and your family the best of health.

Nancy W. Dickey, MD
President, American Medical Association

The American Medical Association

Lynn E. Jensen, PhD, Chief Operating Officer
Robert L. Kennett, Senior Vice President,
  Publishing and Business Services
M. Frances Dyra, Director, Product Line Development

Editorial Staff

Angela Perry, MD, Medical Editor
Christopher Winslow, MD, Pulmonary and Critical Care
  Medicine
Patricia Dragisic, Managing Editor
Mark Ingebretsen, Senior Editor
Marlene Brill, Writer
Barbara Scotese, Editor
Laura M. Barnes, Editorial Assistant

Acknowledgments

Ellen Barish Blum
Linda Cocchiarella, MD, American Medical Association
Janis Donnaud, Literary Agent
LaMorris Perry, MD, Pediatrics
Rolin Graphics, Inc., Minneapolis

Contents

Introduction

Asthma is an illness that affects millions of people around the world. Over 14 million people in the US have asthma. Of that number, about one third are children under age 18. And these numbers are on the increase—up from 10 million in 1990. Treatment of asthma in the US costs billions of dollars each year. In 1990, the cost of lost productivity due to missed school days among children with asthma was estimated at $1 billion. The debilitating effects of asthma can severely limit lives—and, in extreme cases, end them.

In the past, asthma was seen almost as a disability. That is not the case today. With the proper, long-term treatment and the necessary preventive measures, the characteristic symptoms of asthma—shortness of breath, wheezing, tightness in the chest, and a cough—can be controlled. Nearly every person with asthma can expect to become free of symptoms. But for that to happen, the person requires careful and diligent diagnosis and care from a physician. As a person with asthma, or as a parent or guardian of someone with asthma, you will want to learn more about what triggers asthma, how best to treat it, and how to prevent attacks *before* they happen.

The *American Medical Association Essential Guide to Asthma* was written with this goal in mind. Included in the book are thorough explanations of what happens in the body during an asthma attack and the wide array of substances in food and in the environment and in our own bodies that can trigger an attack. The book explains how asthma is diagnosed, which kinds of doctors treat asthma, and what other diseases sometimes mimic symptoms of asthma. The book provides a wealth of specific instructions on what changes you should consider making in your environment and lifestyle in order to prevent or minimize asthma attacks. The chapter on treatments presents an up-to-date wrap-up of all medication and nonmedication treatments available, including alternative treatments such as biofeedback.

This book explains how to create a detailed plan for asthma emergencies when regular treatments do not work. A number of lifestyle issues are discussed, including the impact emotions have on asthma (they can make attacks worse but do not cause them), whether to exercise (yes, with precautions), pregnancy with asthma, breast-feeding if taking asthma medications, and how to help children with asthma. To assist you and your family, the book includes a list of common asthma myths, common questions and answers about asthma, a list of asthma-related resources, and a glossary.

Asthma is a serious illness, and medical science still has not come up with a cure or even a complete picture of its cause or causes. But with the proper treatment, medication, and prevention, you can gain control over your symptoms and live a healthy and fulfilled life. We hope this book helps you in your journey toward health.

1

Struggling for Breath

Four-year-old Sophie had a cold and tenacious cough, as she often did these days. Her father wiped her stuffy nose, tucked her into bed, and read her a story until she nodded off to sleep. Thinking all was well, he finished his chores and went to bed. Around 3 o'clock in the morning, he and his wife awoke to sounds of a loud barking cough. They raced into Sophie's room to find her pale faced and wheezing between the fitful barking sounds. As they rushed her to the hospital emergency department, Sophie's father wondered how a cold could make his little girl so sick. He never imagined the cause was asthma.

Fourteen-year-old David was helping his family by shoveling a thick blanket of snow from the driveway and sidewalks. The previous night's blizzard had resulted in subzero temperatures today, but David was warmly dressed. David attacked the snow vigorously. After about 20 minutes, though, David felt winded. He stood still, coughing and gasping, trying to catch his breath. A sickening feeling washed over him, and it continued for 30 minutes after he came in and sat down. David felt embarrassed by the incident and was relieved when his parents decided to take him to the doctor. Neither David nor his parents ever suspected his problem could be asthma.

Fifty-year-old Janet was getting ready for bed. She had spent a long day cleaning in her basement, which had become mildewed after a flood. Something caught in her throat, making it hard for her to breathe. She coughed and choked, then went for a drink of water. When that didn't work, she blew her nose, thinking mucus from a persistent nasal drip prompted the surprise attack. Nothing eased the choking sensation. Her chest and back felt tight and heavy, so she vowed to be more diligent about her back exercises. For now, however, Janet tried desperately to clear her throat as perspiration beaded on her face. The catch in her throat disappeared in a few minutes, but her inability to take in a full breath lingered. Finally, she drifted into a light sleep, only to awaken exhausted in the morning. Janet did not realize then that her symptoms added up to asthma.

Few people are aware of the many forms asthma can take. At one time, physicians thought people with asthma produced a characteristic wheezing sound. Even the name *asthma* comes from the Greek word *panos,* meaning to pant or breathe heavily. Doctors followed the logic that asthma caused breathing difficulties because blocked airways prevented air from entering the lungs.

Through the centuries, prevailing wisdom dictated a variety of theories for the blockage—some accurate, some not. Physicians connected asthma to a seizure disorder of the lungs prompted by such outside irritants as feathers, smoke, strong perfumes, or animal dander or by psychiatric causes. Treatment focused on reducing a person's symptoms once airways became obstructed. Little was documented about how asthma changed the body's internal systems or the possibility of multiple causes of asthma.

Today, though researchers know more than before, much remains unknown about asthma. An exact cause or cure evades discovery. A few researchers suggest that the different patterns of asthma will one day translate into separate lung conditions. A predisposition to asthma seems to be inherited in some people. Yet, doctors cannot say with certainty why some people get asthma and others do not. The closest thing to an explanation is that certain children and adults have supersensitive airways.

Still, people like Sophie, David, and Janet have reasons to be hopeful. More is known about asthma now than ever before in medical history, and new medications are being developed and made available for hard-to-control symptoms. Although severe asthma can be fatal, the airway narrowing it causes is reversible with proper management. Modern treatment also focuses on prevention, so children and adults with asthma can stop problems before they begin. With symptoms under control, people with asthma can and do lead normal, active lives. The keys to managing your asthma include identifying and avoiding triggers that can cause an attack, recognizing the early warning signs of poorly controlled asthma, and working with your physician to control your environment and use your medications appropriately.

WHY BE INFORMED?

With escalating numbers of diagnosed cases each year, asthma can creep into almost anyone's life. You may be able to name some friend, neighbor, or relative with asthma. Asthma may affect you or someone in your home, and that fact might have drawn you to this book.

As you learn to manage the disease, you may meet people who promote themselves as experts. They may offer their ideas about how you and your family should approach asthma. Most people mean well, and you can assume their guidance is well intentioned. But the advice they give may be based on outdated or inaccurate information. Their recommendations may actually put a person with asthma at risk. This book is designed to help you and your family filter this information.

Except for extreme medical asthma emergencies, many asthma symptoms appear more subtle—unexplained coughing (especially coughing spells in children at night), breathlessness, wheezing. Unless you know someone who has asthma, you may just think you are sick, out of shape, or allergic year-round. Learning about asthma helps you identify whether you or a family member may have the condition.

Asthma has many puzzling aspects. Your asthma symptoms may differ from someone else's and require different treatment. Your symptoms may also wax and wane with the seasons throughout the year. Being attuned to the changes that are likely to occur in your disease can help reduce the frustration that can come from trying to handle so many variable factors.

Along the health-care highway, there are many potholes: quack treatments, dangerous or ineffective medications, and insensitive or unaware health-care providers. Obtaining information about asthma lets you know you have options. Information on asthma is available from both the physician's point of view and the patient's. The knowledge you gather from this book gives you the tools to help yourself.

Once you are armed with information, you can take a more active role in your own health care. If you are uncomfortable with a diagnosis, get another opinion. If your medication seems to be hurting you rather than helping you, request a change. Learn to become your own best health-care advocate.

WHAT IS ASTHMA?

Asthma is an inflammatory disease in which the airways in your lungs become both hyperreactive and hyperresponsive to irritants. *Hyperreactive* means your lungs are more sensitive than most people's and may become inflamed (swollen) when exposed to such irritants as cold air, cat dander, tobacco smoke, or grass. *Hyperresponsive* means your body overreacts to the irritants by tightening the airways and filling them with mucus. Narrowed airways interfere with the movement of air in and out of the lungs, making breathing difficult.

What differentiates asthma from other lung diseases is that asthma symptoms rarely occur continuously. Instead, they come and go in attacks or episodes. Unlike other lung diseases that respond poorly to treatment, asthma symptoms are reversible with proper medication.

The length of an attack depends upon the person and reason for the flare-up. Episodes can be acute, or sudden, or they can build gradually. Asthma can also be chronic, meaning symptoms surface on and off for years.

Although most people with asthma develop it before age 5, asthma can develop at any age. About 25 percent of new asthma patients are older than 40, with 10 percent over age 65. Some asthma symptoms improve or worsen over the years. Episodes in childhood can disappear for years, only to return in adulthood. Studies following children with asthma into adulthood found that those with more severe asthma in childhood experienced more severe asthma as adults. Children who still show symptoms during puberty are unlikely to outgrow their asthma later in life.

Six factors contribute to childhood asthma's continuing into adulthood:

- Disease starting when the person is younger than 2 years
- Allergy as the main trigger
- Frequent attacks
- Ongoing symptoms
- Wheezing, coughing, and other symptoms that suggest hard-to-control asthma
- Presence of nasal polyps (growths in the lining of the nose)

The bad news is the condition rarely goes away. The unpredictability of attacks triggered by a windy pollen-filled day or the perfume of a stranger can be stressful. The good news is that the narrowing of the airways caused by asthma can be reversed. Asthma usually leaves no permanent damage if recognized early and treated effectively, and it does not lead to more severe lung disease. Moreover, asthma can be controlled with early diagnosis and a treatment plan that involves your active participation.

Types of Asthma

Dorland's Illustrated Medical Dictionary for doctors identifies more than 40 types of asthma. Most of these refer to various substances or behaviors that may trigger symptoms. But your doctor may use the terms *extrinsic* or *intrinsic* when discussing your asthma. This breakdown means that some forms of asthma are more often associated with sensitivities to substances in the environment than are others.

Extrinsic asthma refers to attacks that are triggered by exposure to identifiable substances, such as mold spores or dogs; these substances are referred to as triggers. Usually, extrinsic asthma begins before age 30 and may be related to a family history of allergies. At one time, doctors thought that most people under 30 years old outgrew asthma. However, research found that symptoms reappeared later in adulthood in 75 percent of those studied. Sometimes, the same allergies or different ones emerged after long symptom-free intervals. Your physician can help you explore your sensitivity to troublesome triggers.

Intrinsic asthma refers to attacks that occur even though no identifiable triggers can be found. Attacks appear unrelated to seasonal changes or the presence of common allergy-causing agents. Allergy testing, if completed, does not identify any environmental triggers. Although intrinsic asthma can begin at any age, more cases of asthma that begin in adulthood fall into this group. One theory states that unexplainable asthma may be a response to infections, particularly viruses in the lower respiratory tract, that are difficult to identify. After an initial asthma episode from illness, less severe infections may contribute to further attacks. Thereafter, these adults may have fewer periods without symptoms.

Doctors look for the same symptoms with either type of asthma. They realize that asthma symptoms come in different combinations and varying intensities. A diagnosis of asthma follows careful study of these common asthma indicators:

- Shortness of breath
- Wheezing, whistling, or other noisy breathing
- Tightness or aching in the chest
- Persistent cough that lasts more than a week, or coughing attacks after exercise, laughing, crying, or yelling
- Difficulty taking a deep breath
- Excess mucus that will not clear
- Unexplained interrupted sleep, often occurring about the same time each night and resulting in shortness of breath
- Reduced stamina, sometimes to the point where you avoid certain places, such as the beach, or activities, such as gardening

The Impact of Asthma

Although the reasons are unclear, cases of asthma are on the rise worldwide. The National Institutes of Health (NIH) reports that more than 100 million people worldwide have asthma. This global problem touches people of all ages and in every country. In the US, asthma is a leading cause of missed school days, work time, and recreational events. Asthma affects about 12 million people in the US, or 5 percent of the population, and numbers are increasing. Even with improved diagnostic procedures and new medications, the number of cases has increased 34 percent since the mid-1980s.

Asthma is the most common chronic illness in children. Researchers claim that between 7 percent and 10 percent of the youth in the US have chronic breathing problems. Boys under age 10 are twice as likely to develop asthma as girls. Some studies suggest that the higher rates are due to males' having narrower and more flexible airways than females. This difference in physical features, rather than sex alone, may make boys more susceptible to airflow problems before age 10. After age 10, the airway diameter and length ratios for both sexes tend to be equal. The incidence of asthma in boys and girls balances by puberty, with females taking a slight lead into adulthood.

Asthma results in more hospital and emergency department visits for children than any other reason. One report cites 10 million missed school days and 200,000 hospitalizations each year for children alone.

Research suggests various factors that may contribute to the dramatic increase of childhood asthma:

- Increased survival of premature infants with underdeveloped lungs
- Rising numbers of childbearing women who smoke, which increases the likelihood of low birth weights and diminished lung capacity
- Growing numbers of families living in poverty with children who may have greater exposure to polluting substances (such as secondhand smoke from adults' smoking) and along with reduced access to insurance and medical care

Asthma affects all races. In the US, however, children of color are more likely to acquire asthma and breathing complications.

The death rate for African Americans with asthma is six times higher than for Caucasians. Latin Americans are experiencing similar increases in asthma.

Heredity is important to the development of asthma. Evidence gathered from countries around the world, however, suggests that environment and social conditions also play critical roles in determining how widespread and severe breathing problems will be. Studies document that children living in industrial areas or in run-down neighborhoods are at greater risk of developing breathing problems.

New cases of asthma are on the rise in adults, too. Nationwide, death rates due to asthma, though still low, are increasing. In 1996, almost 5,000 Americans died from asthma, a 44 percent rise since 1983.

Medical costs in the US alone increased more than $2 billion from 1985 to 1990 and continue to rise. In addition to medical costs, the practical costs of asthma care, including lost school and work days and quality of life, are astronomical.

Yet, asthma costs more than money and time. Asthma symptoms and emergencies take an emotional toll on the strongest individuals and families. People who feel sick from even the mildest asthma may reduce or avoid activity and limit their normal lives. Daily medication schedules, doctor visits, and constant planning to stay away from asthma triggers can be draining. Add dealing with the inconvenience, stresses, and misconceptions about asthma, and the disease can be overwhelming—unless you understand your asthma and how to control it.

2

Anatomy of an Asthma Attack

Asthma is a disease of exhalation, not inhalation. Researchers know that what makes people with asthma uncomfortable is not that they cannot inhale enough air, but that obstructed airways prevent them from exhaling the air already in their lungs. In fact, autopsies on patients who died of asthma complications have revealed lungs full of air.

Constricted airways trap air in the lungs. This trapped air eventually blocks fresh air from entering the lungs. Mucus produced in the airways further contributes to decreased airflow. What doctors once thought was a problem of inhaling enough air has now turned out to be difficulty in exhaling enough air.

What does an asthma attack feel like? Take a deep breath and hold it for a few seconds. Try to breathe in more air without exhaling first. Do you feel a full, choking sensation? Is your breathing shallow? Add the possibility of mucus clogging your airways and coughing repeatedly to clear the fluid. Are you getting an achy or panicky feeling? These are some of the stresses an asthma attack can cause. What actually happens inside the body when you breathe?

INSIDE THE LUNGS

Healthy Lungs

When asthma makes breathing difficult, the problem is in the airways of your lungs. These two organs are part of the respiratory system that allows you to breathe. The entire system includes your nose and mouth, trachea (or windpipe), and bronchi (or connecting tubes) nestled inside your lungs.

The lungs maintain several important functions. One is to inhale air containing oxygen, which provides fuel for the body's tissues. Another task for the lungs is to exhale carbon dioxide, a byproduct of the tissues at work. Normally, air flows freely in and out of the airways, affording a healthy balance between the two gases. These activities are critical to sustain all the body's vital organs, including the heart and brain.

The Airways

With routine breathing, air goes through a network of airways. Air usually enters the body through the nose. Here the air meets cilia, tiny moving hairs that line the airways. Cilia keep mucus flowing in the nasal passages and filter the air before passing it through the pharynx (or throat) and trachea. Air travels into a series of bronchi that grow smaller as they extend into the lungs. The tubes are wrapped in muscle. The inner lining of the tubes contains mucous glands and various cells. The insides of the tubes are lined with cilia. Bronchi look similar to branches of an upside-down tree, spreading from the trunklike windpipe into each of the two lung cavities.

The Bronchiole Network

As the bronchi stretch deeper into the lungs, they subdivide into smaller bronchioles. A pale, thin membrane known as the bronchial mucosa lines these bronchial tubes. Mucous glands, which keep airways lubricated with watery mucus, are embedded within the many layers of bronchial lining. Harmful substances stick to the mucus and are propelled out of the lungs by the movement of the cilia. Mucus production is one way your body helps fight infection.

The outer walls of the bronchial tubes are wrapped with smooth muscles that can loosen or tighten. This movement controls the size of airway openings, permitting air in or out of the bronchioles. When muscles are loose, airways remain wide open, and air can pass through without effort. When you exhale, muscles tighten. This narrows the airway, allowing you to let air out. Usually, you have no control over this muscle action. Automatic reflexes govern whether muscles contract or relax.

Alveoli and Capillaries

Deep inside the lungs are millions of tiny balloonlike air sacs called alveoli. These sacs surround each bronchiole like bunches of grapes on a stem. The alveoli provide an environment in which the exchange of gases takes place. Oxygen from inhaled air passes into the bloodstream through small vessels, called capillaries, within the sacs.

At the point when air enters the bloodstream, capillaries contain low levels of oxygen and high levels of carbon dioxide. With each breath, the thin capillary walls allow oxygen to migrate into the bloodstream and carbon dioxide to leave. Blood vessels carry the oxygen-rich blood from the capillaries back to the heart, where it is pumped to the rest of the body, and carbon dioxide is exhaled through the airways.

LUNGS WITH ASTHMA

Asthma interferes with the movement of air in and out of the lungs by narrowing the airways. Exactly why this happens is not fully understood.

The most common feature of asthma is inflammation (swelling) of the airways. Doctors have focused their treatments on the connection between inflammation and asthma since the mid-1980s. That is when researchers developed fiberoptic bronchoscopes, which are thin tubes with lights that extend inside lungs. These instruments allowed doctors to view the lungs (and take samples of airway tissues) of people with chronic asthma. From these observations, they concluded that airway inflammation never goes away, even with mild asthma. Their conclusion was to focus treatment on reducing inflammation.

Inflammation, or swelling, is usually the body's response to injury or infection. The last time you cut yourself, your entire body went to work fighting the invasion. Arteries dilated, pumping more blood to the wound. Cells from surrounding tissue rushed to the site, and the skin around the bruise swelled. Specialized cells released fluid to fight infection. Inflammation signaled the beginning of the healing process. When the healing process was complete, the inflammation resolved.

In asthma, however, inflammation continues and can be damaging. You breathe in something that bothers your lungs; then, as in the healing process for a cut, cells within the airway lining are stimulated to fight off the culprit. But these cells release harmful chemical substances that cause a buildup of watery mucus within the lining. In addition, the lining reddens and swells, lessening airflow through the bronchioles. The result is blocked breathing that indicates asthma.

Anyone can experience airway tightening in reaction to irritants, such as cleaning fluids or cigarette smoke. In someone with asthma, the airways are hyperreactive; that is, they overreact, or as some doctors say, become "twitchy."

ELEMENTS OF AN ASTHMA ATTACK

• **Muscle spasm.** Muscles on the outer layer of the bronchi contract, causing the airways to narrow: a bronchospasm. Tightened muscles block airways, restricting the movement of air. Depending upon the degree of airway narrowing, which differs for each person with asthma and with the severity of the attack, the characteristic breathing difficulty, wheezing, and coughing result.

• **Excess mucus.** Inflammation due to asthma can produce excess mucus. During an asthma attack, glands secrete large amounts of thicker-than-normal mucus. Protective mucus clumps together in the airways. Mucus buildup can further narrow the bronchial tubes by partially blocking the passageway, which further hinders breathing.

Increased amounts of mucus can also form plugs that clog very small airways. During an asthma flare-up, some people try to clear their airways by coughing up what seems to be a single mucous plug. But people who have excessive mucus tend to produce many plugs. Consequently, they may have a continuous irritating hack. If left untreated, mucous plugging can prolong asthma episodes and increase the risk of infection.

• **Coughing.** Coughing is the body's way of getting rid of excess mucus in the airways. Coughs result from pressure buildup in the airways that suddenly explodes with a rush of noisy air. When secretions become too thick for cilia to handle, the body coughs to remove the unwanted substance. Dry coughs are the product of extra-thick mucous plugs or bronchioles so blocked that the mucus cannot be removed. Sometimes, nose and sinus drainage irritate airways, producing a nagging cough.

• **Wheezing.** Wheezing is considered to be a trademark of asthma. It results from a forceful rush of air pushing through narrowed airways. The surge of air causes vibrations that make the wheezing sound. Sometimes, however, airways can be so narrowed that the air flowing past a blockage is not sufficient to produce a wheeze. In very severe attacks, the absence of wheezing is a worrisome sign.

Anyone with severe, acute asthma has airway inflammation during an episode. Physicians report that people with chronic asthma have symptoms of airway inflammation all the time. Eventually, uncontrolled inflammation can destroy airway tissue and continue to alter how the lungs work. The results are airways that are permanently obstructed because the continued inflammation scars and alters the bronchial walls. Once this change occurs, the airways do not respond to common treatment. This is why medication to reduce airway inflammation is so important. It prevents airways from becoming permanently obstructed.

• **Fatigue.** Breathing with asthma can tire out the body. It is work just to keep trying to take in enough air. Try breathing through a straw to get an idea of what it is like. Untreated asthma can wear you down.

THEORIES ON THE CAUSES OF ASTHMA

The increase in numbers of people with asthma has spurred the global medical community to more intensive research. Investigations center on newly discovered and existing substances in the body. Attempts to understand mechanisms involved in asthma have resulted in some interesting theories to define the disease more accurately.

Generally, analysis focuses on two systems that work with the respiratory system to influence the lungs: the immune and nervous systems. Many researchers suspect that these control centers may trigger bronchial asthma for some people. They also provide direction for developing treatment and possible prevention and cure.

The Beta Blockade Theory

The nervous system consists of the brain, spinal cord, and nerves. Their job is to control the body's many functions, including breathing. The brain is the system's command center. It receives and interprets messages from receptors in the sensory nerves that take in signals from the environment. The brain sends the necessary orders back out via the spinal cord and network of nerves.

NERVOUS SYSTEM BRANCHES

The *autonomic nervous system* controls the involuntary processes of blood vessels, organs, and other parts of the body. The two main branches of the autonomic nervous system are the sympathetic and parasympathetic nervous systems. The sympathetic nervous system prepares the body for action by quickening the heartbeat and stimulating other parts of the body. The parasympathetic nervous system acts in the opposite way and has more control during sleep. These two systems work like a teeter-totter to balance the body's functions. In the lungs, the parasympathetic system signals the bronchial tubes to react by tightening or constricting. At the same time, the sympathetic system stimulates the bronchial tubes to relax or open. With healthy lungs, the two systems coordinate to maintain open airways, and air flows in and out effortlessly.

In the asthmatic lung, the balance may be tipped toward the parasympathetic system. The imbalance results in narrowed bronchial tubes and asthma symptoms. At one time, the parasympathetic system was thought to be solely responsible for airway sensitivity. Recent studies, however, indicate that although the system is definitely involved, it is not the major reason for inflammation in asthma.

RECEPTORS

Nerves communicate with each other by secreting chemical messengers called neurotransmitters. Each branch of the nervous system produces a different neurotransmitter. The parasympathetic system generates a substance called acetylcholine, and the sympathetic neurotransmitter gives off epinephrine, or adrenaline. Scientists continue to study the importance of these chemicals in bronchial muscle tone. Medications that reproduce the effects of these neurotransmitters are critical to managing asthma.

Three types of sympathetic receptors each process and transmit signals differently. These receptors are known as alpha, $beta_1$, or $beta_2$. Their job is to control all body functions, particularly blood pressure, heart rate, and bronchial tube openings. Alpha receptors carry impulses to raise heart rate, tighten bronchial muscles, and increase mucus production. Although alpha receptors affect the lungs, their role seems less critical in asthma.

$Beta_1$ receptors influence the heart muscle, increasing heart rate and blood pressure. $Beta_2$ receptors, the most relevant for asthma, relax bronchial muscles and lessen mucus production. Research supports the theory that some people with asthma have abnormal beta receptors: the proper neurotransmitters are blocked from reaching the beta receptors; hence, the beta blockade theory. This blockade throws the nervous system off balance, inciting the parasympathetic nerves to overreact and constrict the bronchial tubes. For some scientists, the beta blockade theory explains why asthmatics show symptoms after exposure to nonspecific triggers, such as viruses and extreme weather changes. What remains unanswered are the questions of how and when beta receptors become defective.

The Immune System: Allergy Theory

Similar to the respiratory system, the immune system has its own network of organs, cells, and glands. These fight to keep the body free, or immune, from invading organisms, such as viruses and bacteria. In asthma, the immune system overreacts to elements in the environment.

The main components of the immune system are the thymus gland, lymph nodes, and bone marrow. These produce two major types of blood cells: red blood cells, which transport oxygen from the lungs to the tissues of the body; and white blood cells, which defend the body against infection. Lymphocytes are a kind of white blood cell. There are two types of lymphocytes: B cells and T cells. T cells (T is for the thymus gland in the neck) release chemicals known as cytokines that kill the invading antigen—a foreign substance, virus, or bacteria that invades the tissues and bloodstream. B cells manufacture antibodies, or immunoglobulins, that flag the invader as the enemy so that the rest of the immune system can destroy it. Antibodies also help the immune system to remember and recognize organisms that have infected the body in the past, setting the stage to fortify the body against future invasions by the same substance. Together, T and B cells defend against incoming antigens.

Bone marrow produces about 1 billion white blood cells a day. At first sign of invasion, these cells release T cells to help defend against the invading organism. Once a T cell meets its antigen, it begins to reproduce and kill the antigen it matches. Meanwhile, cytokines enable B cells and T cells to "talk" to each other. The message may be to identify infection or to signal the B cells manufactured in bone marrow to multiply and begin producing antibodies.

IMMUNOGLOBULIN E

Several different types of antibodies guard against disease. One group, however, evolved into a harmful antibody: immunoglobulin E (IgE). Scientists believe that the IgE antibody once helped people ward off common ancient parasites. Although IgE is not needed today, the body continues to manufacture it.

Most people are unaffected by the presence of this antibody, since only about 1 percent of all antibodies produced are IgE. But millions of people have inherited the genetic makeup to overproduce IgE. In some cases, B cells release up to 20 times the normal amount of IgE. If you make too much IgE, your immune system may overreact to routine substances. Each substance you are sensitive to triggers a different IgE antibody.

Any of these could result in allergies that trigger asthma. Studies found that between 30 percent and 50 percent of a random group of people have high levels of IgE in their blood. Not everyone becomes asthmatic, however, and not all asthmatics have increased levels of IgE antibodies that indicate allergy.

MAST CELLS

When allergens are present, IgE antibodies attach themselves to special cells called mast cells. Everyone has millions of tiny mast cells throughout their body, including in the nose, airways, and skin. Even though mast cells are small, several hundred thousand IgE antibodies can crowd into a single cell.

Each mast cell consists of hundreds of microscopic granules filled with powerful chemicals known as mediators. When an allergen arouses an IgE antibody on a mast cell, the mediators release strong chemicals into nearby tissue. This causes the tissue lining to redden and swell.

Depending upon the tissue site, mediators cause many common allergy symptoms. Mast cell eruptions of mediators in the skin can produce hives. Sneezing and a runny nose can develop. In the lungs, mediators can trigger wheezing, coughing, swelling, mucus production, and muscle contractions that signal asthma. The most well-known mediator is histamine. When you have asthma, part of your treatment plan may include taking an antihistamine medication to counter histamine reactions.

EOSINOPHILS

After mast cells explode with their toxic mediators, a host of other chemicals enter the system. These chemicals send eosinophils to the affected area. Researchers once believed that eosinophils were the body's frontline defense against infection. Their job was to regulate reactions to allergens. However, researchers now conclude that eosinophils seem to be a major trigger of airway inflammation in asthma.

Several studies evaluated the connection between eosinophil cells, allergy, and asthma. Patients were given controlled doses of allergens and researchers monitored their blood and their physical reactions. Eosinophil cells quickly passed through the blood to airway sites, leading to increased mucus production and an asthma attack. If the patient inhaled cortisone medication, a steroid that suppresses the inflammatory reaction, the number of eosinophil cells decreased and bronchi overreaction diminished. Researchers concluded that eosinophils release chemicals that contribute to increased airway sensitivity and can create harmful yet reversible inflammation.

LEUKOTRIENES

Investigations have linked other mediator chemicals to the mechanisms of recruiting body-altering inflammatory cells. Studies show that leukotrienes, another chemical released by mast cells, prolong tightening of airway muscles. A group of medications recently was developed to combat the constricting action of leukotrienes.

ASTHMA TRIGGERS

Asthma symptoms begin when something bothers your lungs. These irritants are called asthma triggers. There are many different types of triggers, some acting in isolation and others working together, that make you feel sick. The severity of your asthma depends both upon how many substances in the environment serve as triggers of your asthma and how sensitive your lungs are to these troublemakers.

ALLERGENS

An Austrian pediatrician, Clemens von Pirquet (1874–1929), first coined the term *allergy* in 1906. He used the term to refer to any foreign substance that provoked the immune system or hypersensitivity. Over the years, however, allergies have developed a disruptive rather than protective image.

Allergic reactions in the lungs play a major role in many types of asthma. In fact, the National Heart, Lung, and Blood Institute (NHLBI) claims that the body's tendency to produce abnormal amounts of IgE in response to foreign substances is the strongest

COMMON ASTHMA TRIGGERS

ALLERGENS

- Foods: eggs, peanuts, wheat, fish, milk, soy
- Food additives: sulfites (potassium metabisulfites) in wine, beer, frozen potatoes, dried fruits, cheeses, processed shrimp; tartrazine (yellow dye #5) in margarine, cake mixes, orange cheese, oranges, soft drinks, medications, candy
- Medications: aspirin and aspirin products (multiple-symptom cold tablets, Alka-Seltzer, Midol, Empirin)
- Molds: airborne spores, mushrooms, yeast products (many breads and coffee cakes)
- Food leftovers more than 1 day old
- Pollens: spring tree pollen, summer grasses, fall ragweed
- Latex: tree protein used in manufacture of medical supplies; protein can cross-react with some foods, such as bananas and kiwi
- House-dust mites

IRRITANTS

- Smoke: cigarette, cigar, pipe
- Perfumes
- Household chemicals: nitrogen oxide from natural gas, liquid propane, wood- or coal-burning stoves; carbon monoxide; carbon dioxide; fluorocarbons in cleaning sprays, hair sprays, insecticides, deodorants
- Home building materials: formaldehyde in particle board, plywood, carpet backing, glue
- Work-related chemicals, metal oxides, fluorocarbon propellant, grain dusts, wood dust, sulfur gases
- Hormones: estrogen and estrogen replacements
- Exercise: burst of extreme activity or sustained activity of more than 10 minutes
- Weather: cold, extreme changes in barometric pressure, windy days with low air quality and with blowing pollen
- Respiratory infection: viruses as triggers, bacteria that worsens asthma symptoms
- Gastric reflux
- Nighttime

identifiable factor for asthma. Surveys have documented that more than 80 percent of children with asthma have allergies as well. These children are more susceptible to other allergic conditions, such as in eczema (dry, scaling skin patches) and rhinitis (inflammation of the mucous membrane that lines the nose, popularly called hay fever). As children age, the percentage of people with atopic, or allergic, asthma declines.

New allergy triggers emerge as technology advances. For example, latex, a protein found in tree sap, has become a major allergen for 10 percent to 15 percent of hospital workers. As more medical products were made from latex, health-care workers began experiencing reactions from everyday activity, such as wearing protective rubber gloves. Fifty percent of children born with spina bifida, a neurologic birth disorder, develop latex allergy because they require so many medical procedures.

Although in most instances, atopic asthma strikes before people turn 35, half the adults with asthma are allergic. For some people, allergies build over years until they become strong enough to exhibit signs of asthma. Sometimes, a change in routine, such as a new job or move to a new neighborhood, can expose you to different allergens that can result in asthma.

Even though the connection between asthma and allergies is strong, not all people who develop asthma have allergies. The exact reason for this is unclear. What has been learned is that the numbers of people with both conditions vary in different parts of the world. Your lifestyle, living conditions, and work environment can contribute to chemical reactions that cause allergy and asthma.

ALLERGIC FAMILIES

Allergy tends to occur in families. People are not born with allergies, however. Instead, they inherit the *tendency* to develop some form of allergy that may result in such symptoms as sneezes, wheezes, or hives. They pass on the tendency, rather than the specific allergy and its reaction, from one generation to another.

Allergic asthma depends upon an interaction of heredity and the environment. Your genetic makeup controls your immune system responses, but your particular environment determines which potential allergens you are exposed to.

For those with an inherited tendency toward allergies, the more you encounter a particular allergen, the greater the likelihood you will develop an allergy to it. The length of these contacts contributes to your becoming allergic, too. In other words, what you breathe, eat, inject, or touch can trigger your asthma. Many allergens are so tiny and lightweight they can circulate in the air for a long time. Sometimes, the smallest specks unknowingly inhaled into the lungs can trigger asthma.

COMMON ALLERGENS

The list of allergens is long. Following are some of the most frequently cited allergy triggers of lung disease.

Foods. Your body cannot live without food, yet many foods you eat could be provoking your asthma. Foods are the primary cause of allergies in infants. Allergic reactions in infants may first take the form of crying, a runny nose, frequent ear infections, or eczema. Children who vomit frequently or who have intestinal tracts that seem very sensitive to food may have a greater tendency to develop asthma. As children with asthma age, other symptoms may appear after eating a new allergen. Eating shrimp may suddenly cause facial swelling and itchy skin, or peanuts may prompt hives. Research differs about the connection between diet and allergic asthma in children and adults. Study results conflict as to the most common culprits for triggering asthma: eggs, fish, milk, wheat, peanuts, and soy are all on the list. Children tend to outgrow hypersensitivity to many foods, such as wheat and dairy products. For some reason, however, allergic reactions to shellfish, peanuts, and other nuts may last for years.

Food additives. Manufacturers often add chemicals to foods and medications to keep them fresh longer. Reports estimate that anywhere from 200 to 20,000 additives are in the foods you eat, including preservatives, flavorings, colorings, and sweeteners. Some cause allergic reactions that trigger asthma. (See table below.)

Sulfites. Sulfites, or metabisulfites, are a group of preservatives that are included in processed foods. Before the mid-1980s,

FOODS CONTAINING COMMON ADDITIVES

SULFITES	YELLOW DYE (TARTRAZINE)
Apple cider and other fruit ciders and juices	Breakfast cereals
Beer	Butter
Cheese	Candy
Dried fruits and vegetables	Cheese
Gelatin products (Jell-O)	Canned fruit
Manufactured potatoes	Cough lozenges
Pickled vegetables and meats	Ice cream
Sausage	Mustard
Vinegar	Potato chips
Wine	Toothpaste

sulfites were sprayed on fresh fruits and vegetables, especially at salad bars. By some estimates, 5 percent to 10 percent of people with asthma report severe attacks from sulfites. The additive may also cause itching, rash, upset stomach, and a life-threatening drop in blood pressure.

In 1986, the federal government established guidelines for sulfites. A partial ban on sulfites was enacted for restaurant and supermarket fresh-salad bars. New regulations required labels that indicated sulfites were added to prepared products. Many processed foods and medications still contain sulfites. Some people with airway sensitivity discover the hard way that even their asthma medication contains sulfites. Instead of breathing better after inhaling medication, their airway tightens.

Food colorings. Tartrazine (FD & C [Federal Food, Drug, and Cosmetic] yellow dye #5), a food coloring in oranges, soft drinks, margarine, cake mixes, candies, and some medications, is a troublesome food additive. Years ago, physicians agreed that certain people react to the yellow dye. Today, they claim to have overstated the problem. Few people report reactions, and those who do say the problems are fairly mild. Still, you may want to read labels for any food additives, especially sulfites, tartrazine, and colorings.

Butylated hydroxyanisole/butylated hydroxytoluene. The chemicals butylated hydroxyanisole (BHA) and butylated hydroxytoluene (BHT) are added to grains and cereal products as preservatives. Their presence prevents absorption of oxygen, which can lead to decay. In humans, the two agents can provoke hives, swelling, and other skin reactions.

Monosodium glutamate. The substance monosodium glutamate (MSG) is added to a variety of foods, particularly in Asian cooking, to season and enhance flavor. But in sensitive people, MSG can cause an asthma attack, headache, diarrhea, sweating, chest tightness, and a burning sensation at the back of the neck and upper chest.

Parabens. Parabens are made into several preservatives found in a variety of foods and medications. They are known to stimulate redness, swelling, and itchy or painful skin in sensitive people. Therefore, be alert to products that contain methyl, ethyl, propyl, or butyl parabens, and the more common paraben, sodium benzoate. And be sure to keep track of any asthma symptoms that follow ingesting any product.

Pets. The number of household pets is on the rise. Recent estimates indicate that 43 percent of US householders own dogs, 28 percent have cats, and 4 percent raise rabbits and small rodents. These domestic creatures are covered with fur or feathers. As they go about their business—such as showing affection by rubbing against your body or licking the back of your hand—pets give off saliva, fur, and dander (tiny flakes of skin). Certain breeds of dogs and most cats shed clumps of fur throughout the year. Sticky saliva holds and spreads dander and fur throughout your house. Animals that explore outdoors bring pollen and mold spores indoors on their fur. Any of these substances can trigger allergic asthma symptoms.

For sensitive people, even the slightest exposure to dander can result in airway tightening. The scenario may be dangerous for a child with allergies who houses rodents in the bedroom or sleeps with a dog or cat. Yet people with asthma may react whether or not the animal is in the room, no matter how spotless the house is. Cat dander is unique among allergens in that it remains in the air for a long time. That is why a person who is sensitive to cats can walk into a house and know a cat is in the home without seeing or touching the animal or coming into contact with anything in the house. In many cases, dander lingers in house dust for about 6 months or longer after a pet is gone. Tiny particles of wool and feather, released from clothes, pillows, or bedding, can also cause allergies.

Molds and pollens. Many people with allergic asthma notice that their breathing symptoms change with the seasons. Some experience more symptoms during the fall. Rainy days make them feel short of breath. These reactions can develop from allergies to molds or pollens. Molds are little plants that flourish in damp, dark places. As they reproduce, they send spores into the air.

Outdoors, mold spores can trigger problems from early spring until cool, damp snowflakes cover the ground. Some farmers find that mold from decaying hay activates their asthma. Some autumn hikers find that wet leaves on the ground that harbor mold can produce symptoms. A windy day can blow mold spores indoors to set up housekeeping. Once inside, mold settles quickly. Spores wind up in the most unexpected places—in your mattress, inside garbage cans, under furniture cushions, or between the carpet and flooring.

Spores also thrive in damp places—bathrooms, basements, and where water leaks. Some live in humidifiers, vaporizers, and even air conditioners, where they contaminate the water supply. This creates a double bind for someone with allergic asthma. Increased moisture promotes growth of mold spores. But dry air can irritate bronchial tubes, stimulating asthma symptoms.

Much like mold spores, seasonal pollens permeate the air. Pollens are particles released from plants as they bloom. They are lightweight, so a gentle breeze can carry them as far as 200 miles. Sometimes, they blow indoors when your windows are open.

Every few weeks during spring and summer, different trees and plants flower, sending millions of pollen particles into the air that cause seasonal allergies and asthma. If you feel especially uncomfortable in early spring, you might be allergic to tree pollen. In late spring, your symptoms may be due to grasses. From mid-August until the first frost is ragweed season. Ragweed is one of the biggest causes of hay fever, a form of allergic rhinitis.

Take heart, however. If the person with asthma in your home reacts to pollen exposures, studies indicate that sensitivity to these inhaled particles wanes with age.

House-dust mites. Dust is everywhere, especially indoors. Where dust accumulates, so do dust mites. Thousands of these microscopic insects live in one bit of dust.

A big problem for humans is the feces mites produce. A sturdy coating of protein surrounds each pellet of feces. This protein arouses allergic reactions. As mites die, their decomposed body parts add to household dust and some allergies.

These minute bugs feed on microscopic flakes of human dander that all people shed daily. That is why they are most abundant in bed linens, where skin dander is most prevalent. High concentrations of mites burrow into pillows, mattresses, and box springs. One mattress can conceal more than 100,000 dust mites. Mites hide in upholstered furniture, stuffed animals, carpets, towels, clothes, and air ducts.

Evidence points to dust mites as being the most common potential indoor allergen and a major cause of asthma worldwide.

Studies correlate infant exposure to higher concentrations of mites with greater tendency to develop asthma as toddlers or pre-schoolers. For youngsters between ages 2 and 6, this sensitivity to dust mites shows in skin tests.

People in developed countries seem at greater risk from mites. Lifestyle changes that reflect industrialization seem to contribute to risk increase. Modern insulation techniques may be making conditions ripe for dust mites and, consequently, for asthma. New buildings are designed to be energy efficient and tightly constructed. Airtight homes and offices trap higher concentrations of indoor allergens, encouraging the growth of common dust mites.

In addition, people from industrialized nations spend more time indoors. Adults and children who spend endless hours in sedentary activity—glued to work desks, televisions and videos, and computers—increase their exposure to indoor air pollutants and allergens.

Cockroaches. Among some ethnic groups in certain parts of the world, cockroach allergy is more common than dust mite allergy. Before the development of central heating, most cockroach species lived in tropical climates. Widespread central heating allowed several species to move indoors and multiply. Cockroaches leave their eggs, droppings, and decomposed body parts, all of which trigger airway sensitivity in some people.

Scientists have already discovered components of three different cockroach species in house dust. Like dust mite remains, cockroach remains are difficult to eliminate. Even after cockroaches seem to be gone from apartments and offices, their microscopic leftovers can linger for weeks.

Irritants

Some lungs react to certain substances in the air enough to trigger asthma. Yet, allergy tests reveal no specific allergies. Perhaps, symptoms appear slowly over several years, or you notice that you feel terrible only at work or when you step into your newly remodeled basement. Your symptoms are not in your head. They are the accumulation from repeated exposure to irritants in our environment.

Tobacco. For the past 25 years, the media and the medical community have focused on the dangers of tobacco. Besides causing cancer and affecting the heart, tobacco smoke contributes to several serious lung diseases, including asthma. Despite common knowledge of these health risks, people continue to pollute their bodies and the air around them by smoking.

Any tobacco smoke is harmful, whether from cigarettes, cigars, or pipes—whether or not you inhale. Cigarettes contain damaging chemicals; these chemicals float through the air as smoke, irritating the eyes, nose, and lungs in healthy people. When unsuspecting people have chronic nasal problems or asthma, exposure to smoke can be hazardous.

Cigarette smoke is a major irritant at home and the workplace. Almost anyone with asthma has some reaction to smoke. Lungs in people with asthma are prone to overreact after smoke stimulates sensitive receptors in the airways. These receptors incite muscles surrounding airways to tighten, resulting in an asthma attack.

The effects of passive smoking on nonsmokers are significant. The findings of one recent study suggested that smoking may stunt fetal growth. Studies show that newborns whose mothers smoked during pregnancy have the same nicotine levels as adult smokers. Mothers pass the toxic chemical onto their offspring through the connected bloodstreams. Studies further claim that these babies spend their first few days in nicotine withdrawal, as if *they* were addicted to the chemical.

Infants and children exposed to cigarette smoke develop more respiratory problems. There is evidence to suggest that continued exposure to tobacco smoke contributes to the development of asthma in early childhood. As adults, those who are in contact with smokers and have asthma require more treatment. People exposed to secondhand smoke are also at a greater risk of developing lung cancer and coronary artery disease.

The US Food and Drug Administration (FDA) has sought to exert stricter controls on the tobacco industry, seeking jurisdiction over nicotine as a drug and over cigarettes and smokeless tobacco as drug delivery devices. The FDA is also seeking to prevent the marketing and advertising of tobacco products to children. Some of the proposed controls were still being appealed in Federal District Court as this book was being prepared. New federal legislation instituting new controls over the tobacco industry was also still under consideration by Congress.

Perfume. Did you ever cough, wheeze, or feel your chest tighten after an overperfumed person sat in front of you at a theater or joined you on an elevator? That might mean your lungs overreact to perfume or other odors. Reactions to odors are difficult to monitor, since you usually have no control over what someone else wears, especially a stranger.

Combustible substances. Combustion—the process of burning—releases gases as the substance burns. Products of combustion known to be airway irritants include nitrogen oxide, nitrogen dioxide, carbon monoxide, carbon dioxide, and sulfur dioxide.

Cooking or heating with natural gas, liquid propane, kerosene, wood, or coal produces these irritants, which some people believe may trigger asthma. The results of studies on the subject are not clear, however, and the matter remains controversial.

If your home has gas heating and cooking, make sure the furnace is properly ventilated and that the gas stove has an external vent.

Formaldehyde and other household chemicals. Some people believe that a chemical called *formaldehyde* can cause asthma. Formaldehyde is a gas that irritates the lining of the eyes, nose, and lungs when inhaled. A formaldehyde solution is used as a preservative in shampoos, medications, cosmetics, cigarettes, and even some processed foods. Formaldehyde is also used in manufacturing plastics, wrinkle-free clothing, and building materials, such as particle board, plywood, pressed board, fiberboard, carpet backing, glues, and foam insulation. When these materials are new, a small amount of formaldehyde gas escapes. (How much formaldehyde escapes over time is not known.) The levels of formaldehyde that escape, however, are very low. The question remains whether household exposure to very low levels of formaldehyde is sufficient to worsen asthma. More studies are needed.

Any household chemical gas and odor can trigger respiratory problems. Paints release damaging isocyanate. Cleaning sprays, deodorants, hair sprays, and insecticides have the potential to trigger bronchial sensitivity if they contain fluorocarbon propellants. Compounding the problem is that only about 50 percent of indoor air in insulated buildings circulates with fresh air outdoors. Stagnant and polluted air stays indoors for a long time. Since people in industrialized countries spend up to 90 percent of their day indoors, minimizing indoor air pollution is critical.

Keep records of anything that bothers your airways. Your doctor will want to know.

Occupational Asthma: Work-Related Triggers

Almost any job poses some environmental hazards. With asthma, the problem focuses on the many harmful agents released into the work environment that are inhaled into the lungs. Not all workers exposed to trigger substances develop airway inflammation, however. Only those who have an inborn tendency to lung sensitivity acquire asthma.

In occupational asthma, a worker displays symptoms after exposure on the job to a trigger substance. As contact increases, so does the possibility of lung disease. In a few instances, symptoms disappear when contact with the workplace trigger ends. For most work-related asthma, however, the condition is there to stay. Workers who already have allergies or who smoke are at greater risk of developing occupational asthma. The National Asthma Education and Prevention Program reports several symptom patterns with on-the-job asthma:

- Symptoms improve during days off or on vacation, particularly if the person is taking off 1 week or more
- Symptoms develop within 1 hour or directly after contact
- Symptoms hit 2 to 8 hours after exposure (the more common pattern)
- Symptoms do not appear until nighttime

Because of workers' compensation claims, sensitivities to workplace triggers are the most researched causes of asthma. More than 250 troublesome substances have been isolated as triggers so far, and more appear with each worker complaint. Only a few of these allergens, however, are regulated by the government.

Workers in industrial and agricultural jobs are at greatest risk for occupational asthma. Some of the most potent irritants are hard metal dusts, such as silica, asbestos, and talc, which are used in mining and refineries. Fumes from fluorocarbon propellants and oxides of such metals as copper, zinc, manganese, and iron are also on the long list of agents that provoke lung disease. Since the health-care industry has required that personnel wear protective gloves, more health-care personnel have discovered latex allergens leading to airway sensitivity. As additional research into airway irritants becomes available, the numbers may grow.

The table "Irritants in Occupational Allergies" (see next page) lists some of the most common occupations that involve contact with asthma triggers. Many triggers are known allergens; exactly how other triggers cause airway sensitivity is unclear.

Office workers in insulated office buildings with central air-conditioning systems may never find the source of their symptoms. Fewer than 40 percent of people who feel sick on the job ever discover exactly which pollutant to avoid.

Medications

Prescription and over-the-counter medications can cause sudden asthma episodes. One of the worst offenders is a common pain reliever—aspirin. Studies suggest that between 4 percent and 28 percent of adults with asthma find their breathing more labored after taking aspirin and aspirin-related products. Percentages of individuals who are sensitive to aspirin increase with age and severity of asthma. Most people first notice symptoms in their thir-

IRRITANTS IN OCCUPATIONAL ALLERGIES

OCCUPATION/INDUSTRY	IRRITANTS
Animal worker, veterinarian, laboratory technician	Animal dander, urine proteins
Baker	Flour, amylase (enzymes that convert starch to sugar)
Beauty shop worker	Persulfate, fluorocarbon propellants
Electrician	Colophony (pine resin for soldering)
Farmer (triggers differ with type of farm)	Soybean dust, poultry and storage mites, indoor ragweed, grass pollen, wood dust
Food-processing plant worker	Meat tenderizer, coffee bean dust, tea, shellfish, egg proteins, amylase
Health-care worker	Disinfectants, formaldehyde, sulfathiazole, chloramine, latex, psyllium
Factory worker	Aluminum fluoride, antibiotics
Military, soldier	Mustard gas (sulfur or nitrogen mustard), lewisite (arsenic-containing agent)
Painter	Toluene diisocyanate
Postal worker, bookbinder	Glue
Refinery worker	Vanadium, platinum salts, chlorine gas
Shipping dock workers	Molds, insects, grain dust
Textile worker	Cotton, hemp, flax dust
Welder	Stainless steel fumes, chromium salts, nickel sulfate
Woodworker, carpenter	Wood dust

ties and forties. Once the lungs react to aspirin, the sensitivity appears lifelong. Although the reason is unexplained, a large percentage of these people experience nasal polyps (growths) that chronically obstruct their nasal passages.

Similar reductions in lung function occur from other nonsteroidal anti-inflammatory drugs (NSAIDs) such as ibuprofen and some other pain relievers such as acetaminophen (in higher-doses only). Mostly, these drugs reduce pain and inflammation from such common ailments as arthritis and headache. Some also contain aspirin. Medications are not considered allergens because the reaction has little effect on IgE antibody levels. Researchers are not sure whether people with reactions to aspirin-type drugs always had a sensitivity or the drugs triggered the asthma.

One group of medications called beta blockers can cause airway tightening, leading to bronchospasm. Beta blockers are often prescribed to treat glaucoma, high blood pressure, migraine headaches, and heart disease. Beta blockers work by blocking the beta receptor sites in blood vessels and the heart. Beta receptor sites receive certain neurotransmitters, or chemical messengers, sent by the nervous system. Beta blockers block the beta receptors from receiving the message. Unfortunately, they also block the beta receptors in the lungs, and the missed chemical message can narrow the airways. The chemical reaction is different from an allergic reaction, and sensitivity to beta blockers is not an allergy.

Some people are allergic to penicillin; taking penicillin will trigger asthma symptoms. If you have breathing problems from penicillin, you may also develop hives after eating foods in which small amounts of penicillin are present. Some farmers give their cows penicillin, which is absorbed in milk and meat.

Whether or not you have asthma, be alert to all reactions from medications, especially those you are taking for the first time.

Hormone Changes

Although the relationships between hormonal changes and asthma are still unclear, changes in your level of hormones may trigger asthma. The number of girls who develop asthma at puberty is growing. The ovaries start manufacturing large amounts of estrogen at puberty. A higher incidence of asthma among women continues through reproductive years.

Many women report that their asthma worsens when they menstruate. Research suggests that menstruation alters the body's water and salt balance and changes bronchial muscles and smooth muscles. A few studies concur that premenstrual hormone changes stimulate airway narrowing. One animal study suggests that estrogen restricts airflow through bronchial tubes. More research is needed to discover how and when hormonal changes during the menstrual cycle affect lungs and asthma symptoms.

Similarly, the impact of birth control pills and hormone replacement therapy (HRT) during menopause is being questioned as a potential asthma stimulant. A Harvard team surveyed 23,035 women in the Nurses' Health Study, and doctors found that asthma was twice as prevalent among women who took hormones for 10 years or more during and after menopause.

A connection between asthma and pregnancy exists. About 1 of every 100 pregnant women experiences asthma symptoms during pregnancy. Many more report allergic reactions. For women who have asthma and become pregnant, symptoms for one third will improve, one third will stay the same, and one third will worsen. Usually, women whose symptoms worsen during pregnancy are asthmatics with more severe symptoms. There is no evidence that pregnancy provokes asthma, however.

Exercise-Induced Asthma

Exercise is known to trigger asthma symptoms in some people. Between 70 percent and 90 percent of people with chronic asthma experience symptoms from exercise at some time. Many people who also have hay fever find their only asthma trigger is exercise.

Any burst of exercise or sustained exercise can trigger asthma flare-ups. Reactions can be immediate or delayed, sometimes up to several hours later. *Exercise-induced asthma* refers to airway changes following activity that distinguish it from chronic asthma. With chronic asthma, symptoms can surface any time in response to one or more triggers. However, with exercise-induced asthma, the trigger is more obvious. Symptoms appear when you exercise and can persist for several hours after activity ends.

The exact cause of exercise-induced asthma is unknown. One explanation centers on the loss of warmth and moisture from your airways during exercise. One function of your nasal passages is to warm and moisten the air you inhale before it reaches your lungs. As you exert yourself, larger amounts of air are moving in and out of your lungs, and it becomes more difficult for your nasal passages to warm the air effectively. If the air outside is cool, your airways can cool as they give up heat and moisture to the air you inhale. This process occurs regardless of whether you have asthma. However, after the exercise stops, people with asthma warm up their airways four times faster than people without asthma. Some researchers think that this represents a swelling in your airways. The same type of swelling can occur if you have been outside in the cold without wearing gloves and you immediately wash your hands in warm water after coming inside. The redness and swelling you feel on your hands is very similar to what happens in the lungs of people with asthma.

Airflow problems from exercise result in coughing, wheezing, and shortness of breath. At first, wheezing may not be evident, because exercise stimulates increased production of epinephrine, which can mask the earliest symptoms. Difficulties usually begin 10 minutes into strenuous activity, or within minutes after stopping.

Exercise-induced asthma can occur at any age but is most common in children and young adults. Up to 40 percent of children with seasonal allergies have greater than normal reactions to exercise. Sensitivity is worse during spring and fall when outdoor gym classes and play expose youngsters to pollen.

Many adults may not want to believe that their breathing problems mean asthma. They may instead choose to think that they are out of shape after an episode following minimal activity. Or they assume their symptoms come because they are performing extreme exercise. While exertion can cause fatigue, it seldom results in wheezing, chest tightening, and airflow problems.

A number of famous athletes have asthma and are still able to compete. Asthma triggered by exercise rarely becomes so severe that you need to stop exercising completely, and exercise provides many benefits to your heart, circulatory system, muscles, and even your mental health. Your physician may prescribe taking an inhaler medication (see Chapter 5) 15 minutes before exercise;

this can often decrease the severity of symptoms. Once you stop exercising, continued use of the medication can allow asthma symptoms to fade. Usually, symptoms resolve themselves after about 30 to 60 minutes. If you know you have asthma and you find you are avoiding exercise, you may need different treatment; work with your doctor on this.

Weather

Some people with asthma claim they can predict weather changes better than can meteorologists on news programs. They notice their symptoms worsen or disappear with fluctuating barometric pressures and sudden extreme shifts in temperature. Chest tightening and excess mucus production may warn of high humidity, thunder- or snowstorms, and freezing temperatures.

Cold, which seldom limits airflow with other lung diseases, is a major trigger for many people with asthma. Airway muscles tighten in cool, dry air. The muscles may not relax until temperatures rise again. Even eating cold ice cream can cause muscles to constrict. Hyperventilation (rapid breathing), such as that which occurs after exercise during a cold spell, increases the risk of airway tightening by forcing the body to inhale more cold air than many asthmatic lungs can handle.

Swedish researchers examined 42 cross-country skiers who competed internationally. None had been previously known to have asthma. To everyone's surprise, the study showed that more than half the athletes had asthma. That was 10 times the rate in Sweden's population. The researchers concluded that continually breathing freezing air for many weeks led to asthma.

Summertime can be equally problematic, particularly in certain geographic regions. Dirt, gas, and vapor from smokestacks and vehicles hang over cities in hot, humid air. Outdoor pollution, especially in warm climates, has been known to increase airway sensitivity and heighten allergic reactions.

Two main types of outdoor pollution are industrial smog, such as sulfur dioxide, and photochemical smog, which combines ozone and nitrogen oxides. Some physicians are cautious about implicating these and other environmental pollutants as asthma triggers. But the findings of several studies confirm the relationship between pollutants and asthma, particularly when nitrogen oxides, acid aerosols, and ozone are involved. One German study compared the influence of air pollution on developing asthma and allergies. Researchers collected data about symptoms of children from two cities: Munich, a populated city with heavy automobile traffic, and Leipzig, a city with dense industrial pollution. Results showed that children from Munich were more prone to asthma and allergy, while those from Leipzig caught more bronchitis, a bronchial infection. Other studies have shown that people who move from the country to urban areas are at greater risk for developing lung disease from outdoor pollutants.

Respiratory Infections

Fever, chills, runny nose, and headache are familiar signs of cold and infection. Most people figure these everyday illnesses are part of life. Young children typically catch between six and eight respiratory infections a year, usually from exposure to other children in child care, play groups, nursery school, or primary-grade classes. However, few people with healthy lungs realize that their respiratory infection could put them at risk for developing long-term asthma.

Bacteria. Colds and infections are caused by either bacteria or viruses. Bacterial infections are not currently believed to cause asthma. Once the presence of bacteria, which cause strep throat or otitis media (middle ear infections), is diagnosed, bacteria respond well to treatment with antibiotics. (Viral infections, however, are not affected by antibiotics.) Nevertheless, people with asthma may find their breathing problems worsen during infection. Harmful bacteria in the ears or throat may stimulate nerve endings at the infection site. In turn, the nerves transmit messages into the bronchial tubes that signal the airways to tighten. The presence of bacteria may also increase mucus production and swell airways.

Viruses. Unlike bacteria, viruses cannot be treated by antibiotics. Fortunately, the infections they produce are usually limited; the immune system takes care of them. Viruses can hide inside body cells, however, where they can cause more damage. What begins as cold symptoms may travel into bronchial tubes, resulting in the excess mucus and swelled airways typical of asthma.

Certain viral infections are known to alter bronchial linings. This leaves airway receptors more open to outside intruders. Viruses are also known to alter nervous system messages traveling to the lungs. Bronchial tubes respond by constricting muscles and narrowing the airways.

Researchers are investigating whether viruses actually bring about asthma. In one study, two groups of children were monitored after recovering from a severe respiratory infection. After 9 years, 35 percent still had airway sensitivity, implicating the infection as an asthma trigger. While more research is clearly needed, most physicians agree that viral respiratory disease may stimulate long-term asthma in some children and adults.

Sinusitis (sinus inflammation). Sinusitis is swelling of the lining of the sinus cavities, which lie beneath the cheekbones, next to nasal passages, above the eyes, and deep inside your head. The swelling can be caused by seasonal allergies, irritants, or chemicals. Sinusitis can cause the sinus passages to become obstructed. If sinus infections develop, the obstructions make them difficult to treat. Pockets of trapped bacteria can hide deep inside your sinus cavities.

The swelling and inflammation in the sinuses translate into pressure and pain, which can arouse nerve endings connected to the bronchial tubes. In people with sensitive airways, stimulation of these nerve endings worsens asthma. You may have a sinus infection if you are experiencing:

- Unexplained headache between your eyes
- Pressure or sensitivity under or around your eyes, on the sides of your nose, or on the sides of your head
- Long-term, unexplained stuffy nose
- Long-term, unexplained plugged ears

Gastric Reflux

For some people, the lower esophagus sphincter, the muscle that holds food in the stomach, functions poorly. Stomach acid from partially processed food backs up into the esophagus. Adults call the burning they feel heartburn because the sensation occurs in the chest near where the heart is located. Sometimes, acid seeps up into your mouth, leaving a bitter taste and perhaps threatening to cause vomiting.

Gastric reflux can worsen at night. As you lie down, undigested stomach fluids creep back into the esophagus. At times, you may feel like something is going down the wrong pipe, the windpipe, and this causes coughing. Sometimes, though, the only symptom may be coughing or wheezing.

Gastric reflux is fairly common. When it recurs often, however, the acid in your food pipe can irritate the vagus nerve (part of the autonomic, or involuntary, nervous system). This irritation can lead to a nerve reflex in the bronchial tubes that triggers symptoms of asthma. Doctors are unsure about whether gastric reflux actually causes asthma. They do agree that heartburn is more common—three times more common—in people with asthma.

Stress and Anxiety

Before we developed our current understanding of asthma, one theory held that asthma was the body's way of communicating emotions. Today, the medical community agrees that emotions and mental disorders do not cause asthma. In other words, *asthma is not in your head.*

However, there is evidence to indicate that strong emotions may arouse symptoms in people who already have asthma. Extreme bouts of laughing or fear can cause airways to narrow abruptly. Crying or yelling can stimulate nerves to send bronchial muscles the message to tighten airways. If your asthma seems worse during particularly stressful times, activities designed to reduce this stress may lessen your asthma symptoms.

Nighttime

Asthma symptoms are influenced by the time of day. Often, asthma worsens during the night or first thing in the morning. Many people find themselves awakening with a choking cough, wheezing, breathlessness, or chest tightness. Sometimes, the symptoms last a short while. Other times, they persist for minutes or hours. With recurring nighttime asthma, symptoms disrupt sleep that is much needed to carry out daily activities.

Several reasons account for nighttime asthma:

- In sensitive individuals, increased amounts of dust mites and other allergens embedded in your bedding may trigger allergic asthma.
- Levels of certain natural corticosteroid hormones, which play an important role in keeping airways open, reach their lowest point between midnight and 6 A.M.
- Reduced adrenal gland function can decrease amounts of epinephrine (another substance that helps keep airways open) and corticosteroids in the blood.
- The cold of night can lower temperature in the airways and trigger symptoms, as when exercising outdoors.
- Half the people with asthma find that their symptoms intensify within 4 to 12 hours after the first contact with a trigger—a delayed reaction. Thus, a nighttime attack may stem from a trigger encountered earlier in the day.
- The reclining sleep position increases the likelihood of gastric reflux.

Trying to determine what causes your asthma from the list of possible triggers can be overwhelming. For lack of something definite, you might decide that your asthma flare-ups merely happen without cause. But uncontrolled attacks do not just occur: something stimulates your lungs to react. Discovering you have asthma and what triggers your symptoms are important steps toward diagnosing and preventing episodes and more serious lung disease.

3

Diagnosing Your Asthma

Asthma symptoms may develop so slowly in people and surface so infrequently that you may not know something is wrong. If your schedule is hectic, you may prefer to tolerate symptoms rather than take time to seek a medical opinion. Whatever your response to the possibility of asthma, your symptoms will worsen without attention. Moreover, they could turn life-threatening.

The first move must be yours, however. Without an accurate diagnosis, symptoms cannot be treated. You need to see a doctor if:

- Your symptoms interfere with your ability to maintain daily activities

- You avoid or alter activities that you believe trigger symptoms
- You frequently cough, wheeze, feel breathless, or feel chest tightness
- You awaken at night struggling to breathe
- You already know you have asthma but still endure frequent attacks that signal uncontrolled lung disease

CHOOSING A PHYSICIAN

According to the National Heart, Lung, and Blood Institute (NHLBI), asthma is underdiagnosed and undertreated. Part of the problem lies with doctors who do not keep up with developments in the field of asthma; they may misread asthma symptoms or cling to outdated or inaccurate information. As an example, the myth that everyone with asthma wheezes continues to linger even among a small number of professionals. To prove how prevalent the myth is, one study followed several teenagers who were sent to a cardiologist (heart doctor) complaining of chest pains from exercise. Most never wheezed. Their chest pain was initially misinterpreted as heart-related symptoms, though 75 percent eventually received a diagnosis of exercise-induced asthma.

This example underscores the importance of finding the right physician to treat your asthma. Different medications with serious side effects are introduced each year. New studies document asthma triggers and evaluate drug reactions. Your doctor needs up-to-date expertise to integrate this information into the long-term program that works best for you.

Another consideration with asthma is the personal chemistry between you and your physician. Asthma can require numerous, ongoing office visits. Appointments involve a great deal of exchanging and sharing of information. You will want a doctor who is a good listener, cares about you as a person and patient, and knows what to do to ease your symptoms.

Think about how comfortable you feel with your doctor given these considerations:

- Are you relaxed enough with your doctor to answer the many and varied personal questions needed to diagnose asthma and determine whether treatment is helping?
- Is your doctor someone you can collaborate with over the long term?
- Are you treated as a partner in your treatment program?
- Do you trust your doctor's judgment enough to take your medications as prescribed and comply with the overall treatment plan?
- Do you feel secure that your doctor will be available for you should a medical emergency occur?
- Do you understand your physician's philosophy about asthma and treatment? Are you and your physician working together toward preventing your asthma symptoms?
- Will your doctor take time to explain what is happening, answer your questions, and provide information to help you understand the disease better?
- Will your physician provide written instructions about medication dose and timing and inhalant administration methods?

- How will your doctor respond if you do not follow his or her prescriptive directions?

Generalist or Specialist?

Several different types of doctors diagnose and treat asthma. Generally, your pediatrician, family physician, or internist can recognize the early warning signs. Should your illness spin out of control, you may want to consider seeing an asthma expert.

The physician specialists who treat asthma most often are allergists and pulmonologists. Allergists are specially trained in the evaluation of allergic diseases, among which is asthma. Pulmonologists concentrate on diseases of the lung, such as bronchitis, tuberculosis, emphysema, cystic fibrosis, or asthma. To earn these credentials, doctors complete 2 to 3 years of instruction in their specialty beyond standard medical training. Many ear, nose, and throat doctors, or otolaryngologists, now call themselves otolaryngologist allergists and treat allergy and asthma besides performing surgery. Their training, however, does not stress asthma management and monitoring of complicated allergies.

Several studies have assessed the benefits of asthma management by specialists versus general physicians. For individuals with mild asthma, specialists and general physicians proved equally effective. For those with more severe asthma, however, study results overwhelmingly suggest that respiratory-care specialists have the knowledge and focus that benefit patients. Results indicate that people with asthma who work with specialists experience fewer missed work and school days, decreased hospital and emergency department visits, and fewer relapses.

The National Institutes of Health (NIH) Expert Panel Report

recommends consulting a specialist if you experience any of the following:

- Life-threatening episodes
- No decrease of asthma symptoms after 3 to 6 months of treatment
- Nasal polyps, gastric reflux, or chronic sinus infection, which may aggravate your asthma
- The need for frequent treatment with cortisone tablets or syrup
- The need for specific diagnostic tests, such as allergy skin testing, bronchoscopy, or an allergy challenge
- Examinations that produce only confusion over a diagnosis
- Symptoms that follow a clear pattern that indicates allergy
- The need for special help to control environmental irritants or stop smoking
- Severe asthma episodes in a child under 3 years of age
- Asthma triggered by occupational or environmental hazards that require specialized management

Of course, you will continue with your asthma therapy with the physician who best meets your health-care needs. But it pays to call ahead and ask whether your regular physician can diagnose and treat chest disease. In some cases, a specialist can assess symptoms and recommend a program for your general doctor to follow with you. The main thing is to find help before your symptoms worsen.

When You Have Questions

If you have any doubts or questions, tell your physician. There are no "dumb questions" when your health is concerned. Questions about how your asthma is treated are important because they concern your overall health and they help the physician diagnose and treat you more accurately.

Prepare a list of questions to ask before each appointment, just as you write a grocery list before shopping. You will want to know:

- The treatment options
- Advantages and disadvantages of each treatment
- How the treatments are administered
- What you may experience during treatment

If your doctor resists answering, makes you uncomfortable, or answers with information that leaves you unsatisfied, get a second opinion. The chemistry may be wrong between you, or you may question the diagnosis or treatment recommendations. At some point, you may just want independent confirmation that you and your doctor are on the right track. Any of these scenarios is understandable and justifiable.

Before you make an appointment elsewhere, be sure to request a copy of your file and test results. That way, you will not need to repeat tests with the next physician. You may be charged a minimal fee for copying of the files, but you should have access to this information. State laws ensure that files about your health are your own.

If you are unsure where to find a certified asthma and allergy doctor or pulmonary specialist, there are resources available to you. Ask family or friends for a recommendation. Your general physician or the local hospital or medical society can also be a resource. Some hospitals run asthma clinics or offer referral services for their physicians. Locate an acquaintance who knows the physicians in these referrals. If you still need medical help, contact the national asthma-related organizations, such as the Asthma and Allergy Foundation of America (AAFA) and the American Lung Association (ALA), in the Resources section at the back of this book. Many local chapters of these groups can guide you through the physician selection process.

YOUR MEDICAL EXAM

Diagnosing asthma is a joint effort. You present information about your symptoms. Your physician analyzes your observations and the results of his or her physical examination and, if necessary, confirms the diagnosis with tests. A thorough exam begins with a complete medical history. Think of your doctor as a detective who investigates clues to solve your case. A thorough presentation of symptoms may provide enough clues to continue with treatment without further testing. Think about what your answers would be to the questions listed in "Sample Examination Questions" on the next page.

Trying to remember the fine points of a busy day can be difficult. Remembering what happened weeks, months, and years ago can be impossible. One way to jog your memory and help your physician diagnose symptoms is to keep a daily log (see sample page 61).

Prepare a simple list of possible responses that can be filled in quickly and easily. Write down foods you eat, weather, activities, illness and accompanying symptoms, and any asthma symptoms. Maintain the log for at least a week before your doctor's visit. A log may pinpoint patterns in your activities and your body's

SAMPLE EXAMINATION QUESTIONS

- What makes you think you have a breathing problem? Describe your symptoms. Do you have noisy breathing, wheezing, coughing, or chest tightness? If you cough, do you cough up mucus, and if so, what color is it? Are you ever short of breath?
- Can you remember when and where your symptoms first began?
- Do you have other illnesses? Do you have a history of heart problems or other respiratory illnesses?
- How long do symptoms last? Do you feel worse with succeeding attacks? Do you find yourself exhausted or have sore muscles or trouble breathing long after an attack?
- Do symptoms appear any particular time of day or season? Do they take you by surprise? When are they the worst? When do they seem better?
- Do symptoms seem worse in certain places? If so, do they disappear when you leave the location?
- Do you ever awaken at night with symptoms? If so, what time of night? What happens and for how long?
- Do people in your family have asthma or allergies?
- Do you belch often, feel your stomach juices back up, or have a sour taste in your mouth?
- Do you have any allergies? If so, what are they? Did you have allergic reactions when you were young that came and went? Explain them.
- Do you have frequent sinus infections, nosebleeds, postnasal drip, hay fever, or nasal blockage?
- Do you—or does anyone in your household or workplace—smoke? If you quit, how long ago?
- Has your sense of smell or taste been as keen since you noticed breathing problems?
- Is there more stress in your life?
- Has anything changed in your life lately? Have you moved, switched jobs, had a baby, used new perfume or deodorant, or renovated the house?
- Do you have any pets at home? What kind and for how long?
- What over-the-counter and prescription medications are you taking?
- Do certain foods or drinks make you sick? Which ones? How does your body react?

- Have you found any cockroaches at home during the past month?
- Have you had any serious disease in the past year? Have you had the flu, pneumonia, or other respiratory illness? When you experience cold symptoms, do you feel the symptoms tend to go into your lungs?
- What type of heating and cooling systems does your home have? Do you have a wood-burning stove or fireplace? Are your stoves or heaters unvented?
- Has your breathing ever been so labored you went to the emergency department for help?
- Does exercise trigger breathing problems or chest tightness?
- Have your symptoms affected your daily routine? Explain how.
- What is your job environment like? What materials and equipment do you use regularly? Do coworkers have similar complaints?

responses. You may find perfume makes you sneeze or running upstairs causes you to breathe heavier. Your log may help your physician identify whether you have asthma and, if so, what triggers it.

Heredity

One of the goals of taking a detailed medical history is to assess the role of heredity in your disease. People pass characteristics from generation to generation. Message centers inside each cell, called genes, determine specific characteristics of growth, development, and physical features, such as voice quality, eye color, and gender. In particular, genetic makeup regulates development of the brain, which controls respiration and breathing.

At conception, all babies receive genes from both parents. When an error occurs in any of these genes, a genetic disorder may result. Researchers have explored heredity as a cause of several lung diseases, including asthma. They have already discov-

DAILY LOG OF ASTHMA SYMPTOMS

DAY	TIME	REACTION	POSSIBLE TRIGGER	LENGTH OF REACTION
MONDAY				
TUESDAY				
WEDNESDAY				
THURSDAY				
FRIDAY				
SATURDAY				
SUNDAY				

ered one gene that may possibly cause allergy, an important asthma trigger. Researchers are still looking for genetic material that specifically increases airway sensitivity.

Results of studies suggest that allergy and asthma have separate gene markers. However, if you already have allergy, eczema, or other allergic conditions, the risk of developing asthma increases two- to threefold. Most likely, several genes are involved in allergic asthma reactions. So far, findings of investigations that concentrate on the high levels of allergic asthma occurring between twins, and within families, confirm these assumptions.

One study followed four patients who had lung transplants. Two who originally had allergic asthma received normal lungs. Two other patients with different lung conditions acquired new lungs with mild asthma. Neither of the people with lung transplants who gained normal lungs developed asthma. The two who received asthmatic lungs experienced asthma symptoms within 1 week of the transplant. The results suggest that asthma is an inborn disease found in lungs.

People who are newly diagnosed with asthma, particularly adults who are parents, often ask whether their asthma is hereditary. According to these research findings, the answer is yes. At the very least, heredity increases your chances of developing asthma, especially if allergies are involved. Moreover, you may pass on the tendency to asthma to the next generation.

Should allergies and asthma run in your family, the first 2 years of life are critical for your child. Exposure to potential allergens during this time increases the likelihood that your baby will develop asthma and at a younger age. Early contacts also contribute to the severity of your child's asthma.

The genetic tendency toward lung sensitivity may not follow

a direct line. Asthma may skip a generation or surface in other branches of your family. Inheriting an asthma gene does not necessarily mean you will definitely develop asthma. Children have a 50 percent chance of inheriting asthma from one parent with the condition. The risk increases to 75 percent if both parents carry the disease. But heredity may not be responsible for the increasing incidence of asthma worldwide. Experts claim that genes cannot change that fast in one or two generations.

The Physical

During a physical, doctors look for a variety of diagnostic clues throughout the body:

- What is the outward appearance of the head, neck, chest, and skin?
- Is breathing labored? If you are panting or have obvious trouble breathing, this may suggest airway narrowing.
- Can you hear wheezing and coughing? These are common signs of asthma.
- Is speaking difficult? In extreme cases, your breathing problems may interfere with talking.
- Are you anxious or agitated? Anxiety may be the result of rapid breathing from shortness of breath.
- Are there signs of allergy on the skin? Red, scaly skin that itches may indicate eczema, a skin allergy, and possibly signal other forms of allergy as well.
- Do the ribs bow outward? An alert doctor can recognize asthma by the chest's barrel shape. People with asthma force air in and out by using chest and rib muscles. With

time, the chest walls stretch out of shape, assuming a rounded appearance.

After these initial observations, the doctor checks your glands and other parts of the respiratory system. Swelling in the nose, ears, and under the eyes warn of allergy, as do skin eczema and hives. Nasal polyps distinguish potentially more serious asthma or allergy problems.

The main focus of the exam is on the chest. You will be asked to take deep breaths to assess airflow. As you inhale and exhale, your doctor listens with a stethoscope to the quality of your breath sounds. If there is obstruction, the narrowed passages will cause sudden bursts of air or wheezing or coughing. Inflammation and swelling in your airways narrow your bronchial tubes, making it difficult for you to empty your lungs, so you will exhale longer.

Measured Tests

In many instances, the physical and a thorough exploration of your medical history offer enough information for an accurate asthma diagnosis. Most physicians still order tests, however, to confirm the diagnosis, to rule out any complications, and to help evaluate the severity of your condition. The results provide guidelines that are key to determining an effective treatment plan.

Prepare to spend some time in the physician's office, especially your first visit. Depending upon the number of tests, the entire initial investigation could take 1 to 2 hours. The order and type of tests doctors perform vary, and doctors refine test procedures to suit each patient.

BREATHING TESTS

The most critical tests for evaluating asthma measure pulmonary (lung) function. Essentially, pulmonary testing identifies how well you breathe and the performance of the lungs. Pulmonary tests calculate the amount of air you discharge and the rate of discharge during a single breath. From these assessments, your doctor can discern whether narrowed airways are blocking your airflow.

Pulmonary function can be tested in different ways in various settings. Generally, these tests are not difficult to perform or uncomfortable, although repeated deep breaths with asthmatic lungs can be tiring. Some doctors can measure lung function in their offices. Hospitals and large clinics have more sophisticated equipment for measuring airflow. You may be asked to breathe into a long tube connected to a machine. Or you may be placed in a small cubicle with controlled air and told to breathe. These machines connect to computers that record and assess lung function and print the results.

Before each formal testing situation, you may be asked your age, weight, and height. Guidelines for normal breathing are based on analysis of figures obtained from large segments of the population. Your information will be plotted on a continuum that gives average breathing patterns for healthy individuals of your sex, age, and size. Your airflow measurements are compared with the breathing patterns of healthy individuals with your statistics. Two common methods of measuring airflow assess forced expiratory volume and peak expiratory flow.

Spirometry. A spirometer (from the Latin words for *breathe* and *measure*) is a simple machine used to determine how much air your lungs can hold when completely filled (called your vital capacity) and how long and how fully you blow air out of your lungs. The unit of measure is the amount of air forced from the lung in 1 second, which is expressed as forced expiratory volume (FEV).

To use a spirometer, you first take a deep breath, then blow out quickly and keep blowing until your lungs are empty, then inhale a deep breath again. If initial test results indicate abnormal breathing, the technician will ask you to inhale asthma medication. After medication has had time to open the airways, you will be asked to repeat the test. Now the doctor looks for improvement on the readings that indicate reversibility, a characteristic of asthma. If the volume of air or the flow rate improves by more than 15 percent, chances are the medication opened your airways and you have asthma. If your breathing does not improve, the doctor looks into different options.

A lack of improvement does not totally rule out asthma, however. If your asthma is mild, you may have normal spirometry readings between attacks. For severe disease, your lungs may require 1 to 2 weeks of medication to ease airflow obstruction. Airways may be so narrow that you are unable to complete the task. In this case, the technician will try to document and pinpoint the attempts to measure lung capacity, and you probably will be retested later after a round of medication.

Peak Flow Meter. Another device that your doctor may use to assess your lung function is a peak flow meter (see illustration), which measures how fast you expel air from your lungs. This is your peak expiratory flow (PEF) rate, or peak flow. This device is less sophisticated than a spirometer, which provides a more thorough assessment of lung function. A peak flow meter, however, has the advantages of being less expensive, portable, and easy to use.

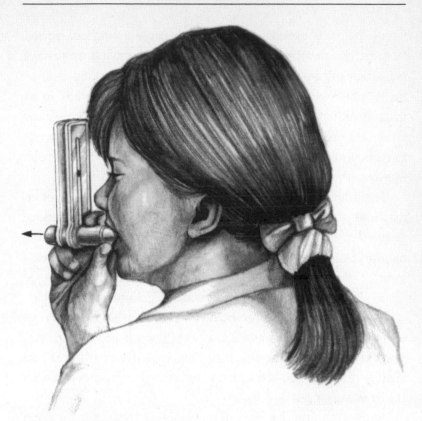

Peak flow meter

The peak flow meter is a device used in the doctor's office or at home to measure your peak flow; that is, the rate at which you can make air flow out of your lungs. To measure your peak flow, take a deep breath and blow as hard as you can into and through the mouthpiece (in the direction of the arrow). Inside the device, the air moves a piston attached to a spring. The piston moves the indicator up the dial to show your peak flow. Through careful monitoring of your peak flow, and by comparing your peak flow to your own personal best and to standard measurements, you and your doctor can determine the severity of your asthma.

Peak flow is especially important because airways narrowed from asthma slow the rate of air leaving the lungs. If your airways are narrowing, you may feel your chest muscles working to force the air out. Your airway muscles are tightening in response to an irritant. As muscles tighten, the lungs become less able to blow air out quickly. By measuring the speed of airflow, you can determine how severe the narrowing has become and, in some cases, foresee asthma symptoms before they appear.

Hand-held peak flow meters allow you and your doctor to diagnose asthma and allow you to monitor your own airflow, away from the medical office or in your own home. Peak flow measures often vary throughout the day and in different situations.

By recording peak flow levels, you can document airway narrowing as it occurs. This can help you identify what triggers your asthma. During serious attacks, a peak flow meter can help you gauge the severity of the attack and help you decide whether you need to call for assistance. Some people can detect asthma attacks earlier using a peak flow meter.

Studies confirm that short-term peak flow measurement helps your physician assess the severity of your asthma. Using the common language of peak flow rates enables you and your doctor to communicate better. Therefore, your doctor may recommend regular peak flow monitoring if your asthma is moderate to severe or unstable. When coupled with a well-written asthma action plan provided by your doctor, peak flow monitoring can help guide you through the treatment of asthma attacks. If your child has asthma, you may benefit from the more definitive assessment of your child's lung function that regular peak flow monitoring provides.

To use a peak flow meter, inhale a deep breath. Blow out as fast and hard as you can into the meter's kazoolike mouthpiece. Blow as if you are trying to extinguish all the birthday candles on a cake in one breath. As you blow, a pointer on the meter moves. The farther the indicator slides down the tube, the greater your peak flow. Your doctor will help you determine your peak flow and what your normal levels should be. Then you can monitor your breathing as part of a total treatment plan. (For more detailed information on how to use a peak flow meter and interpret the results, see page 94.)

Skin Allergy Tests

Allergies are just one of many possible asthma triggers. But asthma and allergy frequently exist together. Allergies usually contribute to asthma in children, and most adults discover some allergies, even if their asthma seems unrelated to these stimulants. Skin allergy testing may help you and your doctor learn what triggers to avoid to limit asthma flare-ups.

Charles Blackley first discovered skin testing in 1873. He scratched some grass pollen into his skin and noticed a small hive develop. Blackley correlated this response to pollen with how his body reacted to ragweed during hay fever season. Over the years, Blackley's basic principles remained unchallenged.

Today, allergists offer three types of skin tests: prick, scratch, and intradermal. Each involves adding small amounts of a given allergen to the skin. The difference is how the allergens are administered. With the prick test, a drop of suspected allergen is placed on the skin and a gadget lightly pierces the skin at that spot.

Scratch tests consist of scraping the skin's surface with a needle and placing the allergens over the scratched regions. Intradermal testing feels closest to getting a shot. A small needle slides under the upper skin layers, where a tiny amount of the allergen is injected. You feel the stick of a needle first, then pressure from the injected allergen. Allergy skin tests are usually given on the lower and upper arms and on the back. Prick tests inject the weakest concentration of allergen and are most often given on the lower arm.

Doctors differ as to which form of skin testing is the best method. Each gives false negatives (stating you do not have an allergy when you do) and false positives (stating you have an allergy, although you do not). Some experts believe that prick testing provides more errors than intradermal. Generally, up to 20 percent of people without allergies obtain positive readings on their skin tests. If you have a positive reaction to an allergen on a prick test, your doctor will most likely check your reaction to the allergen with an intradermal test on your upper arm.

Skin testing covers the most common families of allergens. Each allergen is inserted on a different site that may be marked for later evaluation. Complete analysis could include 47 prick tests on the back for different foods, 30 scratch tests on the lower arm for animals and pollens, and 24 intradermal tests on the upper arm for dust mites, molds, and other allergens the doctor thinks are relevant. Usually, you will receive only about 20 allergens during one sitting.

Two specific skin punctures known as controls are injected in a different location from the other allergens. One is a negative control, a saline solution that produces no reaction. The other is histamine, a known allergen trigger that causes a response in everyone. You may feel itching or burning or see puffy redness or a blister as a histamine response. These two controls provide guidelines for your doctor to compare with your reactions to other potential allergens.

After your regular visit to your allergist, the doctor orders specific test allergens. A technician organizes the allergens and prepares your skin. Once the test allergens are applied, you may sit for at least another 20 minutes. During that time, you may notice a reaction known as a wheal. The wheal can be red with a pale center, and it appears as a hivelike swelling. The size and itchiness correspond with your sensitivity to the irritating test substance. Your wheal may change shape over time, and it will disappear within a few hours.

Skin testing can be time consuming and expensive. If tests are conducted improperly, results can be misleading. Nevertheless, these tests can confirm information that may be difficult to glean through medical history alone. Usually, asthma specialists limit the number of allergy tests on the basis of the severity of your asthma and level of exposure to controllable indoor allergens.

A few people experience delayed reactions to even the smallest amounts of allergen. Hours later, they develop bronchial narrowing that causes breathing difficulty. If left untreated, these reactions can result in increasingly more severe asthma attacks. Contact your physician immediately with information about this or any new development after testing.

Elimination Diets

Many allergists prefer elimination diets to skin tests for differentiating food sensitivity. They worry that some reactions to food go beyond local swelling or itching, especially with asthma. With elimination analysis, the foods you eat and the symptoms that may result are documented in a food diary for at least 2 weeks. Foods that you suspect to be irritants are eliminated. Elimination diets are painless and cost-free. The basic steps for following an elimination diet are as follows:

- Check one food at a time.
- Document in your food diary whether the food triggers allergic reactions.
- Eliminate the foods that seem to trigger allergic reactions. Document daily how you feel without these foods in your diet for at least 2 weeks.
- Start adding back the suspect foods one by one, and note which foods cause you trouble.

Laboratory Analysis

BLOOD TESTS

Under a microscope, stained eosinophil cells leap out of the sample, taking on a brilliant red cast. A test called an eosinophil count measures levels of these cells in the bloodstream. Normally, about 4 out of every 100 white blood cells are eosinophils. But some people with asthma have much higher levels of eosinophils in their blood.

Another blood test calculates the proportion of the antibody immunoglobulin E (IgE) in the body. Blood usually contains changing amounts of IgE over the years. During infancy, IgE levels tend to remain low. They rise gradually for the next 2 to 3 decades. By the time a person is about 40 years of age, the amount of IgE in the bloodstream begins to decrease; the lowest levels are reached when he or she is 70. High IgE levels imply that allergies may be triggering your asthma. An elevated IgE level in infants and young children is one way to predict future allergies.

The IgE measurement has several drawbacks. It does not identify specific allergies, and it cannot disclose whether someone's active symptoms are due to allergens. Although the test is fairly common, it rarely serves as a sole indicator of allergy or allergic asthma.

A group of tests, called RAST (radioallergosorbent test), MAST (multiple allergosorbent test), or FAST (fluorescent allergosorbent test), depending upon the manufacturer, assesses blood levels of IgE for sensitivity to specific allergens. A small blood sample is analyzed to determine how many and which allergens stimulate IgE antibodies. Tests measure for sensitivity to foods, pollens, molds, and animals from a single sample.

Some people with asthma may prefer allergy blood tests because they find one needle stick better than the many pinpricks during skin tests. Others may fear needles, have a skin disorder that will not withstand testing, or know certain skin tests will produce extreme reactions.

Blood IgE tests have several disadvantages, however. Testing techniques are less accurate than skin tests, and results take much longer to obtain. Whereas the effects of allergy skin tests are visible within 5 minutes, blood samples must be sent to outside laboratories and take from 1 to 3 weeks for conclusions, depending upon the test. Expense is another major concern. Blood tests cost about 10 times the amount for skin testing. Companies are working to reduce costs and increase accuracy of results. Until then, most physicians use blood IgE testing as just one option in the diagnostic arsenal.

ARTERIAL BLOOD GASES

To assess the severity of an acute attack of asthma, your doctor may order an arterial blood gases analysis. This precisely determines the concentration of oxygen and carbon dioxide in the blood. Blood gases are usually tested after you have been admitted to a hospital emergency department. This is not a test routinely performed in a doctor's office.

During an asthma attack, inflamed airways block the healthy exchange of gases in the lungs. This causes the gases to be distributed unevenly in the lungs. With moderate to severe asthma, lungs may be working overtime, putting the respiratory system at risk.

This test involves taking a blood sample. More often, the sample is drawn from a wrist artery where both oxygen and carbon dioxide levels can be assessed easily. As with pulse oximetry, arterial blood testing warns of severe asthma that requires immediate, emergency treatment.

PULSE OXIMETRY

A pulse oximeter provides an estimate of the amount of oxygen in the blood. It is a painless, noninvasive monitor that requires a clip being snapped on a fingertip or earlobe. The monitor (oximeter) displays the amount of oxygen it estimates is in your blood.

Because no needle is involved, pulse oximetry is an easy way to estimate the amount of oxygen in the bloodstream, especially in children. It helps doctors predict whether the person will need oxygen supplements. Pulse oximetry can also monitor oxygen levels continuously without interfering with other treatment or with an individual's comfort. Even so, an arterial blood gases test is a more accurate measure of blood gases than pulse oximetry, though it is more invasive. Oximetry is not meant to replace an arterial blood gases test given by a qualified health-care worker. If your asthma attack is severe, your doctor may prefer to obtain a blood gas sample instead of pulse oximetry to assess your carbon dioxide or acidity levels.

SINUS X RAY

When symptoms warrant, your physician may order a sinus X ray. This test determines if sinuses are inflamed or infected, which could worsen asthma symptoms. Sinus X ray identifies the presence of nasal polyps, which are associated with asthma. Nasal polyps are small fleshy growths inside the nose that can cause breathing problems that result in wheezing or obstruct sinuses, causing infections.

Sinus cavities in small children are usually too undeveloped to evaluate accurately. But sinus X ray may be an important tool for diagnosing and managing respiratory problems in older children. Plain X rays of the sinuses can be useful, but a computed tomography (CT) scan of your sinuses provides a more accurate assessment of the anatomy of your sinus cavities.

CHEST X RAY

Although a chest X ray was once a standard tool for assessing asthma, it is usually not used to diagnose this disease. If your physician is unsure that your symptoms are from asthma, he or she may order a chest X ray to determine if another disease is causing your symptoms. Chest X rays are also used to determine whether you have pneumonia, a respiratory infection that may have caused the asthma attack. Spirometry has now replaced X ray for frontline asthma screening.

Asthma Challenge Tests

Many people who suspect that they have asthma may feel perfectly normal between asthma attacks and receive test results that are inconclusive. You may have well-documented complaints that make you and your doctor suspect asthma, but your symptoms are not consistent. This makes your asthma difficult to confirm—and treat. To verify that you have asthma, your physician may suggest performing a challenge test. This test is for adults who demonstrate normal lung function and display little reaction to trials with antiasthma medication. Since having asthma means you have reactive airways, you will be asked to inhale a substance that will cause your airways to react.

Any challenge test is potentially dangerous. There is always the risk that the test may provoke a serious asthma emergency. Even if everyday exposure to a substance normally triggers only a mild response, you may receive a more concentrated dose of the asthma trigger in the test, and more extreme reactions can occur.

The threat of unpredicted delayed reactions is another serious problem. Given these considerations, you should permit only trained specialists to perform challenge tests under controlled conditions. Preferably, challenge tests should occur in a hospital setting. You should expect to reduce your normal activities afterward—just in case a delayed reaction occurs.

INHALATIONAL CHALLENGE

In an inhalational challenge, very small amounts of a substance are inhaled and a breath test (spirometry) is performed. If a reaction does not occur, the amount of the substance is increased and the breath test is repeated. This procedure is repeated until your lung function decreases by 20 percent. A decrease of this amount in all likelihood is due to asthma. The substance inhaled is either a suspected asthma trigger (such as latex) or one of two chemicals: histamine, which occurs naturally in the body, or methacholine, which is known to cause airway constriction only in people with asthma.

EXERCISE CHALLENGE

If you notice that your breathing worsens with exercise, your doctor may recommend an exercise challenge. Spirometry is performed before, during, and after the exercise challenge. You may run on a treadmill or ride a stationary bicycle in a laboratory. A young child or teenager with symptoms may be asked to run freely for a while. If peak flow or FEV drops more than 12 to 15 percent, the diagnosis will likely be exercise-induced asthma.

RULING OUT OTHER CONDITIONS

Your physician may perform other tests to distinguish asthma from other airflow problems. Infants and young children can choke on or swallow food that can go down the windpipe and lodge in the lungs. Some insert small objects into their nasal passages and throat that may lodge in airways. Adults may develop tumors in the airways that must be removed, or they may also accidentally inhale such items as pieces of nuts, broken teeth, or chicken bones into the bronchial tubes. If any of these objects become lodged in the bronchial tree, they can produce wheezing that mimics asthma. Under certain conditions, your physician may recommend bronchoscopy or nasal endoscopy to detect these and other respiratory problems.

Bronchoscopy. On rare occasions, your doctor may suggest bronchoscopy to determine whether a tumor or other growths are lodged in the bronchial tubes. With bronchoscopy, the doctor places a thin, hollow tube, or bronchoscope, through the nose or mouth. The tube attaches to a fiberoptic viewing device or a light and lens. A gentle sedative or local anesthetic allows your physician to insert the tube without too much discomfort for you. The tube extends into the bronchial tubes where mucus or airway cells can be collected for laboratory testing. Forceps can be attached to the end of the tube to remove small, hard objects or thick secretions. Usually, physicians reserve this procedure for cases in which mucus grows so thick or blockage is so severe it is impossible to loosen by less intrusive measures.

Nasal Endoscopy (Rhinoscopy). Endoscopy is a way to see inside the nose and sinus openings. Your doctor inserts a rubber tube into the nasal passages. Attached to the tube is a light at one end and magnifying lens on the other. The view allows your doctor to locate any nose obstruction, sinus blockage, or obstruction in the back of the throat. Usually, the procedure is done without sedation or special preparation, and it may be uncomfortable. But it is a fairly safe and easy-to-perform operation in the doctor's office.

CLASSIFYING YOUR ASTHMA

What does all this testing mean for your asthma? The results of these tests plus your reported symptoms can help your physician identify whether you have patterns of respiratory problems that are associated with asthma. These patterns are compared with guidelines from the National Asthma Education and Prevention Program (NAEPP) coordinated by the NHLBI at the NIH. These guidelines classify asthma into four categories based on the frequency of symptoms or attacks and the results of pulmonary function tests.

Your doctor matches your respiratory profile with one of these categories of severity: mild intermittent, mild persistent, moderate persistent, or severe persistent. Each corresponds to a recommended treatment plan that guides you and your physician in planning the best approach for your asthma. See "Asthma Classification" (next page) to review these categories in list form. If your asthma is classified as mild intermittent, then you only need to take medications when symptoms occur. If you are classified as mild persistent, moderate persistent, or severe persistent, then you will need to take regularly scheduled medications.

Mild Intermittent

Asthma symptoms were once divided into mild, moderate, and severe. But this classification ignored the many people whose symptoms point to asthma but appear only occasionally. Recent NIH recommendations added the category of mild intermittent for anyone with random episodes that occur less than once a week. The person with mild intermittent asthma might experience brief bouts of symptoms lasting a few hours or a few days. Nighttime symptoms surface less than twice a month. When tested, the person's pulmonary function is about 80 percent of normal. Between flare-ups, however, the lungs in a person with mild intermittent asthma appear normal. Therefore, treatment involves a short-acting inhaler that the person uses as needed.

ASTHMA CLASSIFICATION

According to the Global Initiative for Asthma sponsored by the National Institutes of Health, the presence of one of these features is enough to place someone in a category.

FEATURES BEFORE TREATMENT	MEDICATION NEEDED TO PREVENT SYMPTOMS
MILD INTERMITTENT	
Irregular, infrequent symptoms fewer than twice a week	Medication taken as needed
Brief flare-ups lasting from a few hours to a few days and varying in intensity	Extent of treatment depends on severity of episode
Nighttime symptoms fewer than twice a month	Short-acting inhalers
Normal lung function between episodes	
PEF* or FEV† greater than 80 percent but may vary by 20 percent	
MILD PERSISTENT	
Symptoms twice a week but not less than once a week	Daily medication to counter symptoms
Flare-ups may disrupt activity and sleep	Possible long-acting inhaler as anti-inflammatory
Nighttime symptoms more than twice a month	
PEF* or FEV† greater than 80 percent but may vary less than 20 percent	
MODERATE PERSISTENT	
Daily symptoms	Daily medication
Flare-ups disrupt activity and may last days	Inhaled corticosteroid

FEATURES BEFORE TREATMENT	MEDICATION NEEDED TO PREVENT SYMPTOMS
Nighttime symptoms more than once a week	Long-acting inhaler; bronchodilator
PEF* or FEV† between 60 and 80 percent but may vary 30 percent	Short-acting beta$_2$ agonist inhaled daily
SEVERE PERSISTENT	
Continuous symptoms	Multiple medications needed to control symptoms
Frequent episodes	High doses of inhaled corticosteroid
Frequent nighttime symptoms	Long-acting bronchodilator
Limited activity	Oral corticosteroid
PEF* or FEV† less than 60 percent but may vary 30 percent	

*Peak expiratory flow.
†Forced expiratory volume.

Mild Persistent

With mild persistent asthma symptoms such as wheezing, coughing, or breathlessness occur about once or twice a week. Symptoms tend to appear with exposure to cold or exercise and disappear between episodes. Nighttime symptoms interrupt sleep about twice a month. Lung function as measured by peak flow or spirometry is about 80 percent of normal.

Although inconsistent, symptoms occur frequently enough to warrant daily preventive medication. Mild flare-ups usually respond to bronchodilators, medication that works quickly to open airways. Someone with mild asthma rarely misses a day of school or work because of illness.

Moderate Persistent

Moderate persistent asthma displays some symptoms daily. Attacks occur infrequently and can become severe. At least three times a year, symptoms may be severe enough to require urgent, even emergency care. Less troublesome episodes interfere with physical exertion, and nighttime symptoms appear more than once a week. At times, moderate asthma can cause missed school or work time.

Pulmonary tests show only a 60 percent to 80 percent range of normal breathing without medication. Moderate asthma responds to daily medication to prevent asthma symptoms. However, stronger medications may be required to relieve general inflammation and reduce the effects of flare-ups.

Severe Persistent

People with severe asthma experience symptoms such as coughing or wheezing continuously. Sundown brings on symptoms nightly, and people with severe asthma often awaken with chest tightness and shortness of breath. Serious attacks may land them in the emergency department three or more times a year. Episodes requiring hospitalization may erupt more than twice a year. For the most serious attacks, the person may need to be placed on a ventilator machine that breathes for the patient, supplying air through a tube placed through the mouth into the trachea.

Lungs in this category test with 60 percent or less of healthy pulmonary function. Because of the serious risks, people with severe asthma require several daily medications to control their disease.

Most people do not fit into cookie-cutter slots, however, and the same is true of people with asthma. Each person experiences different symptoms with varying severity, and these signs may change quickly. After months of having barely recognizable symptoms, for instance, you could suddenly wind up in a life-threatening situation.

Sometimes, an asthma attack seems to be fading when another attack comes on the heels of the first. This second wave could be more severe than the initial attack. Additional swelling in already swollen airways makes it even more difficult to breathe. If you feel another impending asthma attack, be prepared to seek care to reduce dangerous airway swelling. Do not be surprised if this second wave lingers for days or weeks. Asthma's double assault on the airways leaves them more sensitive to other irritants.

Other Conditions With Asthmalike Symptoms

Adults average about four colds per year, and children catch as many as six to nine. Most come from any one of more than 100 viruses. Medications tend not to act on viruses, so treatment is meant to minimize symptoms and their disruptions.

But when symptoms persist for months, take a serious turn, or hit hard suddenly, perhaps the problem runs deeper than the common cold. Clues that something else is going on include:

- Long-lasting chills
- Achiness
- Fever
- Sore throat or scratchy throat
- Mucus that changes from a clear or cloudy color to thicker yellow, greenish, or gray color

These are additional important signs of when to contact a specialist—someone who can differentiate asthma from other respiratory disorders. If your asthma symptoms refuse to respond despite vigorous treatment, chances are you have more than asthma.

Several chronic airway diseases display characteristics similar to those of asthma. For many, pulmonary function test results indicate comparable reduced airflow levels that may suggest asthma. There is one important distinction, however. With asthma, airflow obstruction is reversible with medication. Impaired airflow from such diseases as chronic bronchitis, emphysema, chronic obstructive pulmonary disease (COPD), and cystic fibrosis resists immediate turnaround. Problems compound, however, when combinations of these conditions coexist with asthma. For example, bronchitis or emphysema can be present with asthma simultaneously.

CHRONIC BRONCHITIS

Bronchitis is an inflammation of the trachea and bronchiole tubes that may lead to wheezing sounds that mimic asthma. Similar to forms of asthma that result from infection, bronchitis is an infection that comes from bacteria, a virus, or inhaling such irritants as cigarette smoke, a chemical pollutant, or dust. The result is acute or chronic bronchitis.

If your head cold turns into a chest cold, chances are you are developing short-term, acute bronchitis. An early warning sign is a deep, dry cough. Without medical attention, the lungs produce a thick, yellowish gray mucus to accompany the cough and head cold. Acute viral bronchitis has no immediate cure. The best thing you can do is rest, drink plenty of fluids, and take acetaminophen or aspirin to relieve general symptoms. (**Warning: do not give**

aspirin to children because they may develop Reye's syndrome, which can be fatal.) Usually, you feel better within 3 to 5 days.

Chronic bronchitis tends to develop more slowly over many years. Illness settles in the bronchial tubes after long-term exposure to irritants and builds up over time. Long-term smoking is the primary cause of chronic inflammation of the bronchial tubes. Smoke damages airway linings and triggers extra production of secretions. Typically, a heavy smoker awakens each day with a cough that can produce a great deal of mucus. The cough never leaves, and mucus production continues to increase.

Since both symptoms interfere with airflow, physicians may prescribe a bronchodilator to relax and expand the airways. If the doctor suspects that a bacterial lung infection is complicating the disease, he or she will prescribe antibiotics. While some improvement comes from medication, airway blockage from chronic bronchitis is not as reversible as with asthma blockage, and the cough does not disappear.

EMPHYSEMA

Emphysema is another lung disease with symptoms that mimic those of asthma. This condition may occur alone or with chronic bronchitis or asthma. A major difference between the three diseases is where they develop. Whereas bronchitis and asthma cause swelling and narrowing of the bronchial tubes, emphysema stems from destruction of the very smallest bronchial tubes that empty into the air sacs, or alveoli.

As emphysema progresses, the alveolar walls become more damaged. Smoking slows the lung's defenses and releases chemicals that cause further inflammation. Gradually, the alveoli lose their ability to exchange oxygen and carbon dioxide. Increased damage causes the alveoli to burst and combine, forming fewer and larger sacs with less surface to exchange the gases.

In time, the person with emphysema becomes breathless. Levels of oxygen fall, which raise blood pressure and strain the heart. Some people try to compensate by breathing faster to inhale more oxygen. As the disease advances, emphysema leads to increased shortness of breath that is irreversible. Eventually, the person with emphysema may require oxygen tanks in order to breathe and may develop a serious risk of respiratory and heart failure.

PNEUMONIA

At one time, contracting pneumonia meant almost certain death. Since the 1950s, however, modern antibiotic medications have greatly reduced the impact of pneumonia and its deadly side effects. Still, pneumonia remains the sixth most common cause of death in the US, and, as for asthma, the number of deaths from it is growing. More males tend to contract the disease, particularly among infants or older adults or when the immune system breaks down from respiratory, heart, or alcohol-related diseases.

Pneumonia is an inflammation of the air sacs, or alveoli, of the lungs that comes primarily from infection, either viral or bacterial. Types of pneumonia differ with the organism causing the disease. Two common types of pneumonia are lobar pneumonia and bronchopneumonia. Lobar pneumonia settles in one lobe of a single lung. With bronchopneumonia, inflammation begins in the bronchioles and migrates throughout one or both lungs, infecting patches of tissue.

Signs of pneumonia include fever, breathlessness, chills, and coughing, often with yellow-green mucus that is sometimes mixed with blood. Breathing causes chest pain from inflamed lung and chest linings. The type of medication depends upon the organism causing the disease. Usually, antibiotics help get rid of pneumonia within 2 weeks. More involved disease can result in respiratory failure.

CYSTIC FIBROSIS

Cystic fibrosis is an inherited disease. Before the advent of modern medicine, children with cystic fibrosis died by the time they were teens. Now children commonly live into their twenties or thirties.

Children and young adults with cystic fibrosis frequently experience many of the symptoms associated with asthma. Common signs of this disease include wheezing, persistent coughing, and excessive mucus. As with asthma, children with cystic fibrosis have a greater tendency toward developing nasal polyps and other respiratory diseases, such as pneumonia. But this is where the similarity ends.

Cystic fibrosis is the leading genetic killer of children and young adults. The abnormal mucus that is a hallmark of the disease becomes so thick it leads to lung blockage, infection, and damage. Cystic fibrosis can also interfere with a person's ability to digest food. People affected can develop chronic diarrhea. Young children often fail to gain weight, despite a good appetite, and they develop clubbed fingers and toes, as well as nasal polyps. The disease affects other organs, eventually shortening the child's life span.

The most common test for cystic fibrosis is a sweat test. Cystic fibrosis stimulates certain glands to produce abnormal amounts of salt, which is released in the body's sweat. High levels of salt (composed of sodium and chloride) indicate a diagnosis of cystic fibrosis. The test involves wrapping a child's forearm with a pad of gauze or filter paper to collect the sweat. A harmless chemical, pilocarpine, and small amount of electricity, stimulate nearby sweat glands. After several minutes, the wrapping is removed and the pad is sent to a laboratory for analysis. If the results indicate cystic fibrosis, the doctor will probably repeat the test to confirm the diagnosis.

Treatment currently is designed to limit symptoms and infection while scientists search for a cure. In 1989, scientists discovered the gene for cystic fibrosis. Researchers are now reproducing healthy copies of the gene with the hope of eventually transplanting it into children with the disease. The hope is for the healthy gene to render the abnormal gene ineffective, leaving the child symptom free. Early testing looks encouraging, but much research needs to be done before cystic fibrosis can be cured. When the day finally comes that several successful transplants have been documented, a cure may be available.

CONGESTIVE HEART FAILURE (CARDIAC ASTHMA)

During congestive heart failure, the heart ceases to pump enough blood to the lungs and the rest of the body. The heart either fails to empty fully with each contraction or is unable to receive blood returning from the lungs. The withheld blood builds up pressure that causes the lungs to fill with excess fluid.

The main respiratory symptom with heart failure is breathlessness. At first, shortness of breath comes after exercise. But over time, lesser amounts of exertion produce symptoms. Symptoms worsen until they are apparent even when the person is at rest.

Occasionally, congestive heart failure can produce wheezing

as a dominant symptom. Although this wheezing is not asthma, it may be confused with asthma if it is the sole symptom. For that reason, wheezing associated with congestive heart failure has been called cardiac asthma. This wheezing, however, is *not* asthma and is treated with medications to lessen fluid retention and to increase action of the lungs.

Other Diseases

A host of other conditions can produce symptoms of lung disease, such as wheezing and coughing, that resemble asthma. Sorting out symptoms that suggest any of these conditions can be complicated. A list of the most common includes the following:

- **Bronchiolitis.** A disease of the lower respiratory tract found in infants and toddlers, bronchiolitis is seen more commonly during winter. Symptoms include low-grade fever, cough, and wheezing that is difficult to distinguish from asthma.
- **Airway abnormalities.** Airway abnormalities may be present at birth but can be removed easily by minor surgery. A stridor, a soft cartilage growth in the throat, is found in some infants at birth. The cartilage causes the child to produce a harsh noise that can sound like asthma. Nasal polyps, as discussed earlier in this chapter, can also contribute to asthma symptoms.
- **Parasites.** Various parasites can invade the body and settle in the lungs, causing infection and breathing difficulties that mimic asthma. A history of foreign travel, earlier parasite infection, or reaction to household pets can offer clues

to this rare condition. Your doctor confirms a diagnosis of parasites by blood tests and stool specimens. Parasitic infections are not common in the US.

- **Congenital abnormalities.** A blood vessel may be pressing on the bronchial tube or there may be heart valve defects, causing asthmalike discomfort.

4

Preventing
Asthma Attacks

Today, most physicians realize the importance of patient involvement in the successful treatment of chronic diseases such as asthma. Studies show that fewer than one quarter of asthma patients actually take their medications as prescribed. Effective physicians have discovered that *involvement* is the key to compliance. Asthma treatment should be a partnership between the patient and physician. As a patient, you provide vital data, and your physician analyzes your observations and responds to your concerns. Together, you develop a treatment plan designed to reduce or eliminate your asthma symptoms.

A large part of achieving your treatment goals and maintaining health involves learning ways to avoid or reduce contact with your triggers. By thinking ahead to prevent symptoms, you establish control over the disease, rather than allowing the symptoms to rule your life.

As yet, there is no cure for asthma. But you can control your symptoms. Asthma usually gives early warning signals, so you have time to act on your behalf. Finding the right plan to follow may take time and patience. Eventually, however, you can learn to:

- Understand the complexities of asthma
- Identify substances that trigger asthma episodes
- Monitor your condition
- Determine your early warning signs
- Intervene early in an attack
- Make lifestyle changes that prevent asthma symptoms from occurring

EDUCATE YOURSELF

Education is power. Once a physician diagnoses your asthma, request material to explain the disease. Ask questions during your visit. Have your doctor define any medical jargon you do not understand. Do not leave the office until you understand your disease and how to implement what you and your physician decide to do.

Work with your doctor to identify your triggers and analyze different treatment options. Make sure you understand what is involved in self-care. Watch someone model the proper use of medication inhalers and peak flow meters. Learn how to recognize when your treatment is not working and when your control over asthma is deteriorating. Your life may even depend upon this knowledge.

If you want more information, contact some of the resources listed at the back of this book. Read other books on asthma for different perspectives. Ask your doctor's office staff for information about asthma support groups in your area sponsored by a local hospital or through the American Lung Association. Discussing asthma with someone who understands something about what you are feeling can help you put your feelings about the disease in perspective. Learning about other people's asthma empowers you to learn more about your own condition and can help give you confidence.

Knowledge and understanding can reduce your fear and increase your objectivity. A diagnosis of asthma may sound scary at first. A severe asthma episode can be frightening. Knowing what your body is going through during an episode and how to deal with your symptoms can be reassuring. Several studies confirm that people who accurately perceive their asthma have fewer symptoms. Conversely, higher death rates and greater numbers of severe episodes have been linked to patients who disregard or misperceive their asthma symptoms.

Look for appropriate help if your child or another family member develops asthma. Find books on asthma that your child can understand. Even young children can grasp information from picture books about asthma that are read to them. Study results show that children who understand their illness and can communicate how they feel can control their symptoms better.

All children go through similar stages of development. Your child with asthma may feel that the illness complicates these normal changes. Introduce your child with asthma to other children with similar symptoms. Youngsters will also feel better if they know a parent can guide them through tough times they may experience. As do adults, children want to know what is happening to their body. Finding others who have asthma makes maturing boys and girls feel less different.

MONITOR YOUR BREATHING

Keep a Journal

Maintaining a log or journal of your symptoms is one way to stay on top of your asthma. You may already be aware of some of your early warning signs of impending attack—wheezing, coughing, fatigue, and breathlessness. Try to always be aware of how your body is feeling so that when you do have an asthma attack, you will remember what happened and how you felt before the attack. Take note of your symptoms, feelings, and circumstances, even if they do not seem related to asthma, and write them down in your journal. By writing down these important signs and sharing them with your doctor during your visit, you are significantly helping your doctor. You are also getting a better and clearer set of warning signs for impending asthma attacks.

Measure Your Peak Flow

Another way to identify an episode before it becomes full blown is to measure your peak flow, the flow of air when you forcefully exhale. Measuring lung function with a peak flow meter can be an important part of your total asthma care. A peak flow meter is an inexpensive, easy method of monitoring breathing, which makes it suitable for use at home. By measuring peak flow regularly, you gain control over silent symptoms that precede an asthma episode and help gauge the severity of the episode.

Moreover, home breathing tests furnish answers to critical questions that guide decisions about your treatment, such as the following:

- How severe is my asthma?
- Which potential irritants trigger my asthma and under what conditions?
- Is my asthma getting worse?
- What families of medicines and which dosages work best for maintaining my regular lifestyle?
- How do I know when to seek emergency care?

Peak flow meters (see illustration on page 67) are available from pharmacies or medical supply stores. Most cost between $20 and $30. Ask your physician or pharmacist for a recommendation. Each meter may read differently, so always perform the test with the same instrument for comparison. You may want to compare readings from your home meter with those on the meter in your physician's office.

HOW TO MEASURE

Anyone over 5 years old who can blow up a balloon can learn to measure his or her peak flow. Ask your health-care professional to model the correct technique for acquiring an accurate reading. Even though there are several types of peak flow meters, the nine steps for using them are similar:

1. Attach the disposable mouthpiece to the peak flow meter.
2. Stand straight and hold the peak flow meter near your mouth and parallel with the floor.
3. Slide the marker to the bottom of the numbered scale before beginning.
4. Keep your fingers clear of the marker line so they cannot interfere with the marker's movement.
5. Breathe in deeply to fill your lungs completely.
6. Seal your lips around the mouthpiece. Keep your tongue outside the hole.
7. Exhale as quickly as you can with a giant burst of air. Remember that the peak flow meter records *how fast* you can blow out, not *how much* you can blow out. Remind youngsters who are measuring peak flow that performing this test is like blowing out birthday candles on a cake with your mouth wide open.
8. Record the numbered results as measured by the marker sliding down the scale. If you cough or have any difficulty, redo the test.
9. Repeat the test twice more. Write the highest of the readings for the three blows in your journal.

The frequency and timing of peak flow measurements depend upon the severity of your symptoms and their stability. Your physician may recommend measuring your flow rate at various times, such as:

- Twice each day
- Before and after inhaling a bronchodilator, if you need one
- At least two or three times a week

If you monitor less frequently, include morning and evening readings on the same day and test before and after using a bronchodilator. Identify whether there is a variation of 20 percent or more, which indicates that your asthma is not under adequate control.

INTERPRETING TEST RESULTS

In the office, physicians compare peak flow against a flow rate chart of individuals with similar age, weight, and height in order to help assess your asthma. Flow is stated in terms of liters per minute. See pages 97 through 99 for tables of flow rate charts for men, women, and children by ages and heights.

AVERAGE PEAK FLOW RATES FOR MEN*
(Liters per Minute)

AGE (YEARS)	HEIGHT				
	60 INCHES	65 INCHES	70 INCHES	75 INCHES	80 INCHES
20	554	602	649	693	740
25	543	590	636	679	725
30	532	577	622	664	710
35	521	565	609	651	695
40	509	552	596	636	680
45	498	540	583	622	665
50	486	527	569	607	649
55	475	515	556	593	634
60	463	502	542	578	618
65	452	490	529	564	603
70	440	477	515	550	587

*Data from Leiner GC et al. Expiratory peak flow rate: standard values for normal subjects. *American Reviews of Respiratory Diseases* 1963;88:644 (from National Institutes of Health. *Teach Your Patients About Asthma.* Publication No. 92-2737, October 1992, p 11).

AVERAGE PEAK FLOW RATES FOR WOMEN*
(Liters per Minute)

AGE (YEARS)	HEIGHT				
	55 INCHES	60 INCHES	65 INCHES	70 INCHES	75 INCHES
20	390	423	460	496	529
25	385	418	454	490	523
30	380	413	448	483	516
35	375	408	442	476	509
40	370	402	436	470	502
45	365	397	430	464	495
50	360	391	424	457	488
55	355	386	418	451	482
60	350	380	412	445	475
65	345	375	406	439	468
70	340	369	400	432	461

*Data from Leiner GC et al. Expiratory peak flow rate: standard values for normal subjects. *American Reviews of Respiratory Diseases* 1963;88:644 (from National Institutes of Health. *Teach Your Patients About Asthma.* Publication No. 92-2737, October 1992, p 11).

The best measurement, though, is to compare your peak flow readings to what doctors call your personal best. Often, individuals with healthy lungs find their peak flow results consistently above or below average predictions for the general population. That's their personal best and their marker for any future respiratory disease. Emphasizing your personal best, rather than average peak flow rates, accounts for the normal variability among people. Your personal best is the highest peak flow measurement on a day when your asthma is under control.

Initially, you may want your physician to help you identify your personal best peak flow measure. Plan to reevaluate your

AVERAGE PEAK FLOW RATES FOR CHILDREN AND ADOLESCENTS
(Liters per Minute)*

HEIGHT (INCHES)	MALES/FEMALES
43	147
44	160
45	173
46	187
47	200
48	214
49	227
50	240
51	254
52	267
53	280
54	293
55	307
56	320
57	334
58	347
59	360
60	373
61	387
62	400
63	413
64	427
65	440
66	454
67	467

*Data from Polger G, Promedhat V. *Pulmonary Function Testing in Children: Techniques and Standards.* Philadelphia, W. B. Saunders, 1971 (from National Institutes of Health. *Teach Your Patients About Asthma.* Publication No. 92-2737, October 1992, p 11).

personal best rating at least once a year after your asthma is under control. As your body changes, so may your asthma. Changes are more obvious with children, who have periodic growth spurts and hormone changes.

If your asthma is not yet stable, a decrease in peak flow can warn you that your symptoms are worsening. Decide with your doctor when your peak flow rate signals that you should contact a professional for help. Besides signaling a breathing crisis, peak flow ratings can identify recurring patterns, such as the following:

• Your peak flow rate significantly drops between nighttime and early morning. This could indicate you need a change in the dosage or the timing of your medicine.

• Your peak flow rate varies greatly, indicating your asthma needs to be controlled. Large fluctuations suggest that you may need stronger medication.

• Your peak flow rate is within your personal best, but you experience sudden flare-ups of breathlessness. This could point to extreme emotions that are causing you to panic or become overanxious. In this case, relaxation exercises or other techniques discussed in Chapter 5 may help.

• Your peak flow monitoring detects consistent drops that signal worsening airway constriction. A decrease of 25 percent indicates a mild to moderate flare-up that can be handled with a bronchodilator to open airways and avoid a more severe attack. But a drop of 50 percent is a signal that you need immediate professional attention, more powerful treatment, and possible changes in preventive medications.

Compare daily variability with your personal best or the National Asthma Education and Prevention Program (NAEPP) asthma severity categories (see pages 80 through 81), whichever is higher. Some health-care professionals explain the categories to children—and adults—with a traffic-light comparison (a color-coded system) that is easy to understand. Peak flow numbers are equally as important, telling you what to do to improve your health.

- Green corresponds with 80 percent to 100 percent of your personal best. This is the zone where the asthma should be. The color signals go, as in go on with your regular activities. If you show no symptoms, take your medicines as usual. You and your doctor may discuss the possibility of reducing ongoing medication.
- Yellow indicates caution. With asthma, yellow indicates approximately 60 percent to 80 percent of your personal best. Yellow also suggests that an acute flare-up may develop soon and that your asthma is not under regular control. You need to talk with your doctor about increasing medication and reevaluating your overall treatment program to ensure symptoms are being managed.
- Red is for 50 percent or less of your personal best. A reading of red indicates a medical emergency. Call (or have someone call) 911 or the local emergency medical services (EMS) system. You need a short-acting bronchodilator (quick-relief medication) immediately and another reading within a short time.

If you feel fine, but your peak flow indicator barely moves, see if your pharmacist or physician will give you another indicator to try. Your peak flow meter may be defective. Should you encounter a defective meter, send it back to the manufacturer and get a replacement.

Peak flow information helps your physician prescribe treatment. Objective readings are particularly important in a medical emergency.

AVOID YOUR TRIGGERS

Perhaps you and your doctor were able to isolate one or more factors that directly trigger your asthma symptoms, or maybe not. Either way, by now your symptom diary and peak flow readings give you some indication about which situations or offending substances contribute to your asthma. You have made a strong start, but there is more you can do on your own.

Becoming involved in preventing your disease helps you avoid possible triggers or actively work to lessen their impact. Particularly with allergy-induced asthma, reducing exposure to indoor and outdoor allergens is important for preventing symptoms. Avoiding triggers over a long period of time leads to decreases in airway swelling and sensitivity. With serious asthma, determined preventive care can keep you from developing permanent airflow damage.

Prevention often implies lifestyle changes—for you, your child, and other family members. Perhaps it means giving up favorite foods, finding different medication, or avoiding certain places. Change may prove difficult to carry out or accept, but the benefits to health and well-being are worth any inconvenience. Following are some suggestions for lifestyle changes that can make a difference for someone with asthma.

Foods and Food Ingredients

Preventing allergic reactions to foods involves more than carefully reading labels. Frequently, labels fail to reveal troublesome substances because they appear under unfamiliar names. See the table on the next page for a list of common substances that may be food allergens.

FOOD ALLERGEN	SUBSTANCES CONTAINING OR CONTAINED IN FOOD ALLERGEN
Milk	Casein, calcium caseinate, whey
Eggs	Albumin, ovomucoid, ovomucin
Soybeans	Textured vegetable protein, vegetable-derived protein
Corn	Grain alcohol, corn syrup, cornstarch, medications bound with corn flour

Tiny amounts of ingredients sometimes do not appear on labels. Products that are completely pure usually state that the contents are "100 percent" of the main ingredient. Without such an indication, you may need to eliminate the food product from your diet. Other hidden ingredients in processed products could provoke an allergic reaction.

A few people find they react to certain foods in the same food family. For example, people bothered by bananas may also discover a sensitivity to avocados. This is known as a cross-reaction. Sometimes, combining two foods causes a different unexpected allergic reaction. Ask your physician about other foods that commonly cross-react with the food to which you are allergic. Check the books about food allergies listed in the Resources section at the end of the book for further information.

Indoor Allergens

Most likely, you spend considerable time indoors. The amount of asthma medication you need may closely relate to your exposure to indoor allergens. Therefore, a good place to begin managing symptoms is at home.

DUST MITES

Dust mites are tiny insects related to ticks (and more distantly related to spiders) that eat human dander (flakes of dead skin). They live in cloth objects inside the home: linens, upholstered furniture, and especially pillows and mattresses. Some people are allergic not to the mites, but to their feces, which accumulate over time. Dust mites are rampant in humid regions, which includes most of the US. Eliminating the dust mite population in your home can be difficult, but there are ways to shrink their numbers. The extra effort you take may provide real benefit.

Dust mites depend upon indoor humidity to live and multiply. Therefore, anything that reduces moisture helps control dust mite colonies. Since mites reside in greater numbers where you sleep, your bedroom is a good place to begin serious mite control.

Here are some indoor precautions:

• Air conditioning removes moisture from indoor air. Studies confirm that in warm, humid regions, such as in Florida or Hawaii, air conditioning also reduces the number of mites.

• Encase your mattress and box spring in allergy-proof, airtight zippered covers.

• Purchase an airtight pillow covering, or plan to wash your pillow weekly.

• Replace down and feather pillows with hypoallergenic fiberfill pillows and mattress pads that also inhibit the growth of bacteria, certain molds, and fungus.

• Wash sheets, blankets, and bedcovers weekly in hot water. Make sure the water is at least 130 degrees Fahrenheit, the temperature required to kill house-dust mites.

• Remove carpets from the bedroom. Vinyl or polished wooden floors limit hiding places for mites. You can lay washable area rugs instead. If removing carpeting is impossible, cover the carpet with polyethylene sheeting that can be attached to the baseboard molding.

- Do not sleep on upholstered furniture. Vinyl, leather, and plain wood furniture harbor fewer mites. Cover upholstered chairs and sofas with plastic to keep the mite population down.

- Hang washable miniblinds, shades, or lightweight curtains instead of heavily lined drapes, which can act as allergen catchers.

- Wash your child's stuffed toys in hot water or deep-freeze them once a week. Try to eliminate or at least limit the number of stuffed objects in your child's room and definitely in bed at night.

- Damp-mop and dust twice a week. You can use any dust-catching product sold in stores, but be alert to airway sensitivity to spray chemicals. Avoid sweeping with a broom in the bedroom. Brooms circulate dust in the air instead of removing it.

- Clean closets, drawers and shelves every 3 months. Dust settles on shelves or creeps into drawers—just waiting for you to pull something out, sending dust mites whirling into the air.

- Wash window screens regularly, especially those that sit in basements or sheds all winter.

- Rid your home of dried flowers, knickknacks, or other difficult-to-clean dust catchers that become mite hideaways. Shelve books and magazines in enclosed bookcases or sealed boxes. Display prized collections behind glass-covered curio cabinets.

Besides residing in the bedroom, dust mites homestead throughout your house. Many of the above recommendations for cleaning bedrooms apply to any room.

Although chemicals are available to rid rooms and furnishings of mites, researchers question whether exposing children and adults who already have airway sensitivity to strong chemicals is an acceptable risk. Refer to the Resources at the back of this book for information about where to obtain these and other products.

COCKROACHES

A recent study identified cockroach droppings and body parts as major allergens that could cause children's asthma to worsen. Controlling cockroaches involves regular, thorough housecleaning. If you find one bug, you can assume the rest of the family is close behind. Wet-mop or vacuum the pepper-looking spots of cockroach droppings on the floor and inside cracks. Seal the cracks you cleaned with caulking or weather sealants, such as silica gel or other silicone-based caulking. Since these products may irritate sensitive airways, you may want to wear a dust mask or ask someone else to apply them.

Seal any potential entries into the house. Cockroaches are able to squeeze between narrow spaces, such as around pipes and wires into the home, surrounding window frames, and under doors. As a precaution, store foods and garbage inside sealed containers, and never leave unwrapped foods on counters. To reduce the number of cockroaches, be sure to:

- Disassemble and clean exhaust fans
- Fix drippy faucets and leaky pipes
- Ventilate humid or stagnant areas where cockroaches go
- Wash dishes before going to bed
- Free drains of food scraps
- Keep food out of rooms where someone with asthma sleeps
- Clean behind stoves and movable cabinets and under refrigerators regularly

- Empty and clean pet food and water dishes soon after your pet's feast and do not leave pet food out overnight. (Pet food attracts insects the same way the food you eat does. If you must leave your pet's food out, place the bowl in a slightly larger bowl filled with soapy water. Bugs find soap offensive and won't cross the moatlike barrier.)
- Clean litter boxes daily
- Wash the area where pet droppings occurred immediately with a damp cloth

Try to avoid using pesticide sprays and bombs. These may irritate your asthma. Instead, select insecticides that are not airborne. You can find nonallergenic pest strips, bait stations, pellets, or boric acid at your local grocery or hardware store. If you must apply an insecticide, ask someone else to spray while you leave the house if you are the family member with asthma. After spraying, air out your home for a few hours to minimize exposure to irritants and wet-mop or vacuum the roach body parts and droppings.

If you live in an apartment building, contact the building manager or landlord for professional assistance in ridding the entire building of infestation. Otherwise, your neighbors' roaches may infest your cleaner apartment, and your efforts will be fruitless.

INDOOR MOLDS

Molds form in dark, moist, and poorly aired places where there is dampness. Like cockroaches, molds thrive in any season. Make sure your basement, kitchen, and bathroom are well ventilated year round. Wash and dry tiled walls, fixtures, and floors regularly with a strong fungicide soap solution. The NIH recommends that people with asthma who live in tropical climates tile the walls in these rooms to prevent water seepage and to lower humidity.

To keep mold at a minimum:

- **Remove or disconnect humidifiers**. If you live in a temperate climate, you may want to add humidity to your home for comfort during dry winters. But you still want to keep your home dry enough to prevent molds and dust mite growth. Ideal levels are between 20 percent and 40 percent humidity. Dust mites thrive in humidity of 50 percent and above.

You can maintain consistent moisture levels in your home using a hygrometer, an instrument that measures humidity in the air, and adjusting your humidifier accordingly. If you plug in your humidifier during winter, maintain consistent humidity by occasionally turning off the humidifier and opening windows. Moisture is naturally added to the air from your body, as well as during cooking.

- **Install a dehumidifier.** In areas of your home with high humidity, such as basements, use dehumidifiers to help to reduce mold and bacteria.

- **Run your air conditioner.** The air conditioner will help reduce humidity and filter large mold spores and yeasts from the air. Regular use of your air conditioner controls humidity and lessens dust mite growth. With air conditioning, your windows and doors stay closed, which reduces the number of outdoor pollens that migrate indoors.

- **Ventilate rooms.** Regular ventilation helps reduce spore density. Exhaust fans in bathrooms and kitchens decrease water vapor from cooking and bathing. They draw out mold spores, especially in homes with central air conditioning. Repair leaks in tile and plumbing fixtures immediately to avoid seepage.

- **Remove leather products, books, stuffed toys, and dried flower arrangements**. Clean them with mold-killing solutions. Molds and dust mites grow on indoor plants, too. Limit these in your sleeping areas, and water them with fungicides every 4 weeks. If plants prove too difficult to clean regularly, give them to someone who is allergy free.

- **Air out objects.** Boots and running shoes stored in closets can be mold breeding grounds.

- **Clean moldy areas.** Use a half bleach–half water solution. If your airways react to bleach, try a mixture of distilled white vinegar and baking soda.

- **Wipe the refrigerator clean**. Use a bleach solution regularly and remove spoiled foods. Empty water pans below self-defrosting refrigerators regularly.

- **Examine wallpaper for mildew**. Mildew is a fungus that grows under moist conditions. If the mildew proves impossible to clean, seal the paper with a nonlatex paint sealant.

- **Spray chemicals that kill mold and prevent regrowth in high-humidity areas.** Bathtubs, sinks, and air conditioners are considered high-humidity areas. You can find the chemicals in hardware stores or in the Resources section at the end of this book. Use pumps instead of more irritating aerosols.

- **Correct water seepage problems.** If your basement floods, inspect the area, fixtures, and furniture carefully to make sure no mold is growing on wood or other surfaces.

Animal Allergens

Any furry, warm-blooded animal is a potential allergen. Even the smallest rodent produces dander, urine, and saliva that can trigger asthma symptoms. All breeds of dog or cat are potential allergy triggers.

The best action you can take to prevent allergic asthma is remove the animal and any feather products from your home. Even after you remove such items, animal allergens stay imbedded in carpets and furniture for months, so you may need to keep cleaning. Apply 3 percent tannic acid in areas with animal dander to reduce contamination.

Giving away a pet can be heartbreaking. If this seems out of the question in your situation, there are steps you can take to lessen exposure to animal allergens:

• **House the animal outdoors, if possible**. At the very least, keep the pet out of your sleeping area. This is important, since your symptoms may worsen at night.

• **Close your bedroom door at all times.** To keep your animal from slipping inside your bedroom, keep the door closed at all times. Install a door lock or latch if necessary.

• **Limit where the pet is allowed to roam**. If possible, remove upholstered furniture and carpets in the areas your pet frequents so that animal allergens cannot collect in them.

• **Wash your pet weekly**. Even cats who usually hate water can grow accustomed to regular baths. If your feline resists at first, wash a small area at a time until the cat accepts full bathing. You can also treat your animal's coat with a spray or solution that cuts down on dander. Ask for recommendations from your animal's veterinarian, the pet store, or an allergy supply company.

• **Wash your hands after touching any animal.**

• **Keep your fur-bearing friend out of the car, where the animal's dander could linger.**

- **Choose a snake or fish for your next pet.** Snakes and fish may not be as cuddly as other kinds of pets, but they lack fur or feathers that trigger asthma symptoms.

Clearing the Air at Home

A wide variety of other potential allergens lurk indoors. Most are invisible to the human eye, but they are sizable enough for your airways to catch them and react. Air cleaning tips include the following:

- **Cover air ducts, particularly to the bedroom, with a dense filtering material**. Filters trap animal dander, mold spores, dust mites, and other tiny particles stirred up by forced-air heating and air-conditioning.
- **Avoid vacuuming if you have asthma**. Even being in the same room when someone else vacuums exposes you to an increased level of airborne allergens. Conventional vacuums gather large particles but permit smaller dust, mites, and molds that easily enter the lungs to escape from the loosely sealed collecting bag. During vacuuming, and for about an hour after, you can encounter more dust than before cleaning began.
- **Rugs and floors need cleaning at least once a week**. If you have asthma, ask someone else to vacuum, and leave your home for several hours. If you must vacuum, wear a dust mask that traps fine particles. Select a vacuum with a powerful suction. Make the vacuum healthier for everyone by adding high-density collecting bags or a high-efficiency particulate air (HEPA) filter for the exhaust air. An alternative is to buy a central vacuum with

a collecting bag that can stay outside the home, such as in the garage. But a central vacuum is expensive and requires that you have storage space outside your home.

• **Steam-clean rugs.** The disinfecting effects of steam-cleaning have been proven to reduce the number of mites in carpets for about 6 weeks. Cat dander, however, is more resistant than mites to heat, and steam-cleaning shows no effect on cat dander imbedded in rugs.

• **Purchase special air filters.** Air filters decrease levels of airborne allergens considerably. Before you buy a costly air filter, however, decide which allergens are critical to remove and whether a filter would make a dent in their numbers. Some allergens are heavy enough to settle onto carpet and furnishings before they can be filtered from the air. For example, dust mites and indoor mold spores fall from the air after 5 minutes, rendering an air filter almost useless. Tobacco smoke and wood smoke, however, linger in the air in high levels, so a filter is useful if a smoker lives in the home. Cat dander remains airborne for hours, so again, a filter is helpful. Depending on the allergen that affects you, you can determine how valuable a filter will be for preventing your asthma.

There are several types of air filters. Some are freestanding with a fan and simple filter, and others attach to central air heating units. In general, most filter systems fail to eliminate enough of the offending particles from the air. Two devices stand out for their effectiveness. A HEPA filter removes most particles, no matter what size. The other system involves electric current; the device is called an electrostatic precipitator. With this filter, a charge zaps the airborne dust particles and collects them on metal plates inside the instrument. This filter is less effective than the HEPA filter, but it can be attached to your central air-conditioning unit. The drawback is the metal plates require regular cleaning.

Before you order any air filter, measure the size of the room where the filter will go. The size of filter you want depends upon the volume of the room. The volume is a measure of the room size and amount of air it holds. No matter what size and type of device you buy, however, air filters never replace regular, thorough house cleanings.

• **Change or clean air-conditioner, ventilation, and heating systems regularly.** Clean the air system often, empty your dehumidifiers and humidifiers often, and change filters monthly. Otherwise, mold, mites, fungi, and mildew collect in these units, forming another home for growing irritants.

TOBACCO SMOKE

The most obvious indoor irritant to avoid is tobacco smoke. At the very least, never permit smoking around you or your child who has asthma, and never permit smoking in rooms your asthmatic child uses. Ask visiting smokers to smoke outside.

When away from home, stay out of confined places where people smoke. Never ride in a vehicle with a smoker. Always request nonsmoking sections at restaurants and nonsmoking rooms at motels and hotels.

If you or a family member has asthma and you smoke, the best alternative is to stop. Study results show that people who stop smoking cough and wheeze less and breathe easier. Just 1 month after stopping, you may experience fewer infections and better lung function.

In theory, ending smoking sounds great. The reality is that

nicotine in cigarettes makes smoking highly addictive, which makes quitting difficult. If you have problems stopping smoking, try weaning yourself from nicotine by replacing tobacco with chewing gum or a nicotine patch. Call the local chapter of the American Lung Association to request *Freedom From Smoking for You and Your Family,* a self-help manual, or videotapes or audiotapes that can help you quit.

You may prefer to follow a prescribed program for quitting. Investigate the many programs for smoke-ending or ask your physician for recommendations. Contact the American Lung Association about joining one of their Freedom From Smoking Clinics. Your life and the lives of your family members demand the effort.

OTHER AIR POLLUTANTS

Besides tobacco smoke, other air pollutants could irritate your asthma. Common household soaps, detergents, and cleaners may bother you. So that you can reduce contact with strong odors and sprays, the American Lung Association recommends that you use a simple mix of natural cleaning products, such as (but not limited to) distilled white vinegar, baking soda, Borax, and Murphy's Oil Soap. Many natural products cost less than ones with synthetic chemical ingredients. You can wash, polish, and deodorize your entire household with greater security knowing that these products will probably not bother your airways.

Even the safest products and most thorough cleaning might still leave your home with airborne pollutants. Try these suggestions for reducing exposure to troublesome irritants:

- Vent your furnace to the outdoors to prevent noxious gases from escaping into rooms of your home.

- Have your heating system inspected yearly for worn-out parts, gas leaks, or other problems that could affect air quality.
- Be careful about the cooking oils and cosmetics you buy. They may not trigger a full-blown attack, but they could make you feel sick.
- Check gas- and wood-burning appliances and oil or kerosene stoves to make sure that flues or ducts are functioning properly to reduce your contact with carbon monoxide, nitrogen oxides, and nitric oxide.
- Avoid wood-burning fireplaces. Ashes and smoke can blow inside the room.
- Ventilate rooms you are painting. Better yet, let others do your painting, repairs, and improvements, and leave your home while they are doing so. Paint, cleaning solvent, and wood finishes release irritating odors into the air. If possible, stay somewhere else overnight until after decorating smells subside. One way to hasten your return is to apply water-based paints that dry quicker than oil-based products.

Avoiding Allergens Away From Home

OUTDOOR AIR

Certain seasons can play havoc with asthma. Pollens (grasses, weeds, trees), mold spores, and elevated levels of air pollution (ozone, sulfur dioxide) probably cannot be avoided completely if you are sensitive to them. But you can limit your exposure to these irritants.

The most obvious way to limit contact with outdoor pollutants is to stay indoors. Close the windows and turn on the air conditioning. Not everyone wants to limit themselves to the indoors, however. Less confining preventive options include the following:

- Be alert to reports that mold and pollen counts are high; remain indoors then. Most weather reports include pollen and pollution alerts.
- Refrain from exercising on high air pollution days. If you must exercise outdoors, choose low-traffic residential areas where pollution is lower.
- Try to travel outdoors early in the morning before ozone and sulfur pollution accumulate.
- Ask someone else to mow the lawn, rake leaves, or cut trees. Mold spores and pollens collect in outdoor organic substances. If you must perform these tasks, wear a pollen mask and bathe immediately afterward to wash pollen and grass shavings from your body and hair.
- Review your vacation plans with a health-care professional. Check whether the season and your destination are likely to aggravate your allergies.

IN THE CAR

Do you experience sudden breathing problems on your way to work? The problem may be your car air conditioner. One study's results revealed that molds causing the greatest sensitivity in allergic people grew in stale water and condensation from automobile air conditioners. People with allergic asthma reported their symptoms worsened in the car, and tests confirmed decreases in lung function after people drove with the air conditioner on.

To avoid symptoms, clean your car air-conditioning system regularly. Contact an auto dealer or repair person for the best way to clean the system thoroughly.

AT WORK

If you suspect that some substance or condition at work affects your asthma, try first to have it verified through testing (see Chapter 3). Determining which substance or substances cause or worsen your asthma may be difficult. You may want to see a physician who has experience in diagnosing and treating occupational asthma. If tests confirm that your asthma developed from exposure to a substance or substances at work, you may need to discontinue all exposure. Discuss your findings with a supervisor or on-site health-care provider. Try to provide creative and fair suggestions for:

- Avoiding the asthma-causing agent
- How the company might provide better ventilation
- Alternatives that the company might investigate, including different manufacturing process or substances that lessen potential dangers for all workers
- Wearing airway protection, such as a dust mask
- Working while attached to a portable respirator or wearing a helmet respirator
- How the company might institute a policy for a tobacco smoke–free environment

Under the Americans With Disabilities Act of 1990, employers are responsible for making workplace accommodations for special needs. This includes employees with respiratory problems, such as asthma. If you offer reasonable alternatives but still encounter management obstacles, suggest that your employer contact the Job Accommodation Network, a toll-free international consulting service that offers job accommodation information. Remind the employer that:

- The company saves money keeping a qualified worker and not training someone new
- Accommodations will enhance your productivity because you can breathe easier
- Your productivity increases when you feel the company supports and appreciates your efforts on their behalf enough to make changes

Point out that these accommodations may prevent future respiratory illness in other employees. Any steps taken to reduce or remove asthma irritants may save money in the long run for potential workers' compensation costs, which vary from state to state. Accommodations may also head off any legal or government intervention on behalf of other affected employees. Reinforce the fact that the law requires employers to make reasonable accommodations for workers with special needs, such as asthma.

If reasonable alternatives are not possible—if, for instance, your only option is to switch jobs within the company and for some reason you cannot do that—immunotherapy (allergy shots, discussed at the end of this chapter) may reduce your sensitivity enough to allow you to work. If the particular allergen or irritant is not susceptible to a course of immunotherapy and no other alternative treatment can be found, you may need to leave your job and find work elsewhere. The damage to your lungs will only worsen. Over time, the damage may leave you unable to work at all.

Keep Your Body Healthy

COLDS AND INFECTIONS

Flu and colds are unavoidable. But you can reduce your chances of getting sick and minimize risks from infection you might acquire by keeping these health practices in mind:

• Eat a balanced diet that has large amounts of high-fiber, unprocessed foods. Avoid foods prepared with additives, such as chemical preservatives and food colorings, that might cause sensitivities.

• Exercise regularly, following your doctor's guidelines.

• Drink 6 to 8 glasses (or more) of water and warm liquids daily to flush out potential allergens and keep your entire body working smoothly. Plenty of water helps to thin mucus, so your airways remain clear and free from buildup.

• Avoid large crowds and people whom you know to have a cold or flu. Wash your hands after being with someone who is sick. Hand washing is an excellent way to avoid the spread of disease.

• Get plenty of rest. Breathing with asthma can be tiring, so you may need to make extra time to rest.

• Take over-the-counter medications that are recommended by your physician. Some nonprescription cold remedies, antihistamines, and cough syrups react adversely with asthma medication. Avoid aspirin and aspirin-related medications that may trigger asthma sensitivity.

• Ask your physician for an annual flu vaccination, especially if your asthma is moderate to severe. Vaccines have been refined to limit unpleasant reactions that once discouraged people from submitting to flu shots.

GASTRIC REFLUX

Heartburn (a burning sensation in the esophagus and stomach), frequent belching, or regurgitation of food into the back of your throat are all symptoms of gastric reflux. As food passes from your esophagus to your stomach, it passes through a one-way valve that prevents backflow. In some people, this valve is malfunctioning, which produces the symptoms. In the 1990s, researchers have demonstrated an association between gastric reflux and asthma. If your asthma symptoms, especially coughing and wheezing, are most bothersome at night, gastric reflux may be a factor contributing to this problem.

If you experience gastric reflux frequently and suffer several nighttime asthma episodes a week, here are some simple suggestions for minimizing the effect of reflux on your asthma:

- Elevate the head of your bed on up to 6-inch blocks or sleep on a wedge pillow to prop up your head.
- Stop smoking; smoking can aggravate digestion.
- Avoid eating and drinking for the 3 hours before you lie down.
- Eat smaller portions of food at each sitting. As you age, your body naturally slows, needing less fuel to keep going. You may find you need to eat more frequently to maintain your energy. Eating smaller meals more frequently satisfies both concerns.
- Eat a balanced diet and avoid foods that leave you feeling unsettled.
- Resist eating fatty or spicy foods and choose drinks without alcohol or caffeine, which can cause indigestion.
- If you take any medication with theophylline and suspect

that gastric reflux could be contributing to your asthma, talk to your physician. Theophylline weakens the one-way valve between your esophagus and stomach, and it may be the wrong medication for you.

- Talk to your physician about other medications, prescription or nonprescription, that could quiet reflux symptoms.

WEIGHT CONTROL

Why your weight matters. Too much weight forces your body to work harder. If you are overweight, your breathing is heavier and your heart pumps more blood to supply extra nutrition to body tissues. With asthma, your body may require more energy to perform the simplest activities. Asthma medications may add to the problem by causing you to retain fluid and gain weight. Plan ahead by watching what you eat to maintain a realistic weight.

Exercise with care. Exercise can improve your energy level, allow for a healthy weight, and help you fight infection. These factors are important to building lung stamina. But improperly performed exercise can produce asthma symptoms and attacks.

Devise an exercise plan with your doctor that gradually increases your energy level and breathing capacity yet prevents asthma symptoms. Fifteen-minute warm-up exercises before your workout can help your lungs adjust to the extra burden of exercise. Symptoms can be minimized by taking two puffs from your bronchodilator before you begin exercising. End exercise with a gradual 15-minute cool-down rather than an abrupt stop.

Stay alert to how you feel during exercise. If you experience symptoms, stop to rest and take medication before the symptoms grow worse. Avoid exposure to allergens, such as pollen, that worsen your asthma. Cold air and low humidity put stress on asthmatic lungs. During cold weather, it is best to avoid outdoor exercise. If you must exercise outdoors, wear a scarf or filter mask to warm and humidify (make moist) the air going into your lungs. Consider indoor exercise when your health is at risk from hay fever pollens and high pollution alerts. (Learn more about exercise and asthma in Chapter 7 and the Resources section at the back of this book.)

A PREVENTIVE TREATMENT OPTION: ALLERGY SHOTS

Certain troublesome allergens are impossible to avoid, yet your asthma refuses to calm down even with environmental controls or use of medication. Or your highly specific job training makes it difficult to transfer jobs. A possible alternative to reduce airway sensitivity, thereby preventing asthma attacks, may be immuno-therapy, more commonly known as allergy shots.

With immunotherapy, small amounts of the diluted allergen are injected into your body. The body's immune system quickly produces substances called antibodies that block an allergic reaction. As you repeat this process once or twice a week for 3 to 4 months, the body becomes sensitized to the allergen. As your immune system reacts less, your allergy symptoms subside.

Gradually, you receive higher concentrations of the allergen until your body tolerates the highest dose without reacting. Your physician may reduce the frequency of shots but continue injecting the elevated allergen dose for up to 3 to 5 years. There may be improvement with 3 to 4 months of injections. Successful immunotherapy results in fewer symptoms and a decreased need for medication to control allergies, such as hay fever, or asthma.

As with any treatment, there are drawbacks. Immunotherapy

may not always work, and it can be costly and time consuming. Your physician will want you to stay about 30 minutes after receiving the shots so you can be observed. Most allergic reactions from shots occur within that time. Usually, health risks are minimal. Mild reactions, such as swelling around the shot, help determine the next allergen dose. More generalized reactions, however, can vary from itching and sneezing to severe asthma attacks. In rare cases, airways close and blood pressure plummets, signaling a medical emergency. That is why only qualified physicians in a medical office should administer allergy shots.

If the correct allergies are covered, immunotherapy may work for some adults and children. Studies report that this preventive treatment reduces symptoms of allergic asthma if the allergies involve animal dander, house-dust mites, pollen, or fungi. But research cannot confirm whether the positive effects last. Weigh the pros and cons of immunotherapy with your physician.

5

<hr>

Treating Your Asthma

Modern medicine has come a long way in understanding asthma and how to combat its effects. New research builds on knowledge, refining strategies, medications, and how they are delivered. As yet, asthma may not have a cure, but nearly all asthma is controllable. Armed with information about your asthma, you and your doctor can develop strategies to counter breathing difficulties.

Medication advances plus your control measures form the basis of your treatment plan. You may also choose to investigate alternative asthma treatments. Most effective plans with traditional physicians, however, involve medications to handle long-range consequences and short-term flare-ups. Your overall treatment should include methods to:

- Reverse airflow barriers
- Stop symptoms from occurring so you feel better

- Prevent serious attacks and the need for emergency care and hospitalization
- Keep asthma from interfering with everyday activities
- Prescribe medicine that leaves no or minimal side effects
- Control symptoms with the least amount of medication

Your physician will probably follow the step approach to prescribing medication that is recommended by the National Heart, Lung, and Blood Institute (NHLBI). The more severe your asthma symptoms, the higher the doses of more powerful medication you will need to take. Medication guidelines correspond with the severity of your asthma. In other words, you and your physician determine whether your asthma is intermittent, mild, moderate, or severe before treatment begins.

Physicians differ in how they prescribe medication on the basis of this step approach. Some treat symptoms with the weakest medications for a given step. If symptoms prove difficult to control, they add stronger medications from a higher step. Other doctors prefer to work from the top down, trying for rapid control of symptoms and then reducing medications to the smallest doses that will be effective. The step concept is important to understand, since you may need to deal with the effects of too much or too little medication.

MEDICATIONS FOR YOUR ASTHMA

Everyone's asthma varies. Your airways react to different triggers. Your symptoms flare on their own schedule and your own symptoms vary. Therefore, dosage, timing, and type of medication must be tailored to your individual needs. That is why so many different forms of medication have evolved. Your medication may be inhaled, taken orally in pill or liquid form, or in emergency situations, injected into your bloodstream.

Unless otherwise indicated, all the medications discussed in this chapter are available only by prescription.

Inhalers

Inhalers are devices that allow you to breathe medication into the lungs. Three popular forms of inhalers include aerosols, dry powder, and nebulizers.

AEROSOL (METERED-DOSE) INHALERS

Metered-dose inhalers (MDIs) rely on a mixture of medication, preservatives, and liquid propellant gas to deliver medicine into your lungs. You breathe in and press the top of the inhaler. This releases puffs of inhaled medications directly into the airways. Some inhaled medications begin to reverse airway narrowing within 5 minutes. Both short-acting and, more recently, longer-acting medications have been developed in inhalant form.

Aerosol medications have some advantages over oral medications. They go straight into the lungs rather than circulate to the heart and throughout the bloodstream before reaching the airways as with pills or liquids. This means weaker medications inhaled directly are able to perform the same job as stronger oral doses. Equally important, inhaled medications reduce the systemwide adverse effects from medicine exposure with oral (pill) forms.

Aerosols are usually handheld, small enough to carry in your pocket, lunch box, briefcase, or purse (see illustration, next page). This puts your medication within easy reach should symptoms occur.

Aerosol (metered-dose) inhaler

Aerosol inhalers, also called metered-dose inhalers, allow you to inhale asthma medicine into your lungs. After inserting the medication dispenser and shaking the canister gently and removing the cap, exhale completely and place your mouth around the mouthpiece. Depressing the medication dispenser releases a puff of medication into your lungs as your inhale.

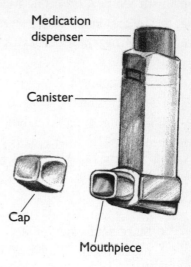

Medication dispenser

Canister

Cap

Mouthpiece

Warning: Because inhalers seem safer than pills, patients sometimes do not discuss possible unpleasant or negative effects of inhaled medication with their physicians. But such adverse effects do happen. Unusual symptoms that do not seem to have a direct cause may stem from your medication. Document your symptoms and how often they occur and review your notes with your physician.

TRIGGER AND BREATH-ACTIVATED INHALERS

Some metered-dose inhalers discharge medication after you press a trigger at the top of the shell. Newer versions are breath activated. When you suck in forcefully, your breath prompts a mechanism inside the inhaler to shoot out a dose of medication.

The two types of aerosols perform similarly. For individuals with poorer coordination or impaired hand function, such as people with arthritis, breath-activated devices may improve delivery of the medication. During severe attacks, however, a lack of air may make triggering the device difficult.

USING YOUR INHALER

Two techniques offer the best control of inhaled medications. One method requires that you hold the inhaler 1 to 2 inches from your mouth. The other entails your placing the inhaler into your mouth. Otherwise, both methods involve the same steps, as follows, that should be followed for best results from your metered-dose inhaler:

- Make sure your inhaler has enough medication. (See the next section, "Knowing When Your Inhaler Is Empty.")
- Remove the cap and position the inhaler upright. Remember to keep the inhaler capped when it is not in use. Otherwise, foreign objects may become lodged in the inhaler and may be accidentally inhaled into your airways.
- Shake the inhaler vigorously.
- Hold your head upright and exhale until your lungs are empty.
- Hold the inhaler 1 or 2 inches in front of your open mouth.
    or
- Place the inhaler in your mouth and seal your lips around it.
- Release the medication as you breathe in slowly but deeply.
- Hold your breath for about 5 to 10 seconds to allow the medicine to absorb thoroughly into your airways.
- Breathe out slowly and relax.
- Repeat the process for as many puffs as your doctor orders. If you are using a bronchodilator, wait 3 to 5 minutes be-

tween puffs. If you are using an inhaled corticosteroid or cromolyn, you do not need to wait between puffs. (These types of medications are described later in this chapter.)

KNOWING WHEN YOUR INHALER IS EMPTY

A major problem with metered-dose inhalers is knowing when they are out of medicine. Running out of medication can be a serious health hazard. You usually cannot see, hear, or taste when the canister is empty or delivering less medication than intended. Sometimes, inhalers feel heavy enough to hold medication but only contain propellant and preservatives. These may leave a strange taste or heavier spray in your mouth, indicating the medicine is out.

Each inhaler has a label that reports how many measured (metered) doses the canister holds. But how do you know for sure when to reorder your medicine? Do you wait until the inhaled medicine tastes different or the canister totally empties to reorder? Neither is a good choice.

For regularly scheduled medications, it is best to calculate the number of days until reordering time. Divide the number of doses by the number of puffs you inhale per day. The resulting figure indicates how many days your medicine should last. For example, if you use 4 puffs twice a day, your daily total is 8 puffs. If your canister contains 100 puffs then it contains enough medicine for 12½ days. You can mark your calendar, or directly on your canister, the date that you need to buy another inhaler.

This system works fine for medication taken regularly on a schedule. But what about the bronchodilator you inhale sporadically? Keeping track of how many times you sprayed is inconvenient. Even when you follow up diligently, your inhaler may still contain less medicine than the label indicates.

The best option is to measure how full the canister is. Remove the shell, and place the canister in a pan or sink filled with water. Watch what happens. If the canister sinks to the bottom, you know it is full. A partially full canister floats halfway down or partly lifts out of the water. When the canister floats sideways on the surface of the water, it is totally empty: time for another prescription.

Note: do *not* immerse inhalers that release a dry powder, such as cromolyn sodium, nedocromil, or budesonide. Submerging these canisters can cause powder residues to form a paste that will plug up the canister, preventing it from working. All other types of canisters can be put in water.

In some cases, the canister merely needs cleaning. To clean the canister, rinse your plastic inhaler and cap, without the metal cartridge, with brisk running water. Dry it thoroughly before replacing the cap and cartridge. Remember to clean the inhaler after each use and to shake it well before every treatment. Otherwise, the inhaler clogs, which inhibits your receiving the prescribed dose of medication. Regular cleaning also prevents your inhaling bacteria with your medicine.

PROPELLANTS

Most current metered-dose inhalers propel medication with chlorofluorocarbons, such as freon. Some people find these chemicals irritate their airways. Also, chlorofluorocarbons harm the earth's upper atmosphere by breaking down protective ozone molecules, and some people with asthma may object to chlorofluorocarbons on environmental grounds. Many European countries have banned freon-pressurized inhalers. In the US, such canisters will be outlawed by the year 2000, although legislators may exempt the ban for medical purposes. Alternate chemicals that do not harm the environment, such as HFC 134, are under investigation.

SPACERS

Your physician may give you a hollow device called a spacer (see illustration) that acts as a bridge between you and your spray inhaler. Spacers attach to different types of inhalers, providing a

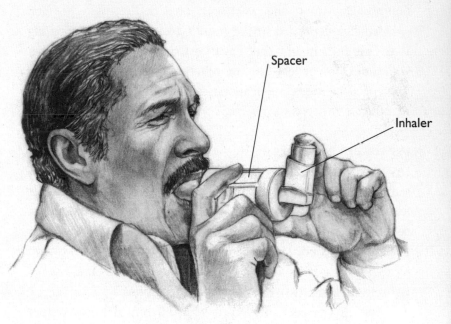

Spacer

Inhaler

Spacer

A spacer is a plastic tube that attaches to your aerosol (metered-dose) inhaler. The spacer momentarily traps the medication as it comes out of the inhaler, making the medication easier to inhale and preventing it from being lost. Spacers benefit people who find it difficult to squeeze the trigger and inhale at the same moment, such as younger children or older adults.

space in which to trap medication so you have more time to inhale. As you inhale, a spacer helps direct medicine into the lungs.

Spacers come in varied sizes and shapes to suit the inhaler. The simplest spacer is a plastic tube that slips into the mouthpiece of your aerosol inhaler. Larger-volume spacers and face mask varieties hold more medication. Flexible masks fit over the nose and mouth, helping children, older adults, and those with coordination problems to breathe easier with inhalers.

Medicine deposited in the mouth area can produce side effects. Spacers help limit this, ensuring that more medicine reaches your lungs. You benefit from more targeted medicine without the side effects of strong medications, such as corticosteroids, in the mouth and throat.

DRY POWDER INHALERS

Dry powder inhalers (see illustration, next page) incorporate the same benefits as other breath-activated inhalers. You do not need to coordinate inhaling with releasing medication. People concerned about the environment prefer knowing they never inhale irritating gas propellants or release them into the atmosphere. More powder inhalers may be brought onto the market as manufacturers seek alternatives to chlorofluorocarbons.

Some dry powder inhalers have a different delivery system from that of metered-dose inhalers. These involve inserting a capsule with medicated, fine powder into the canister. Each capsule usually contains a single dose that equals two sprays of medication, although double doses are available. After inserting the capsule, you turn the canister, which opens the capsule and frees its contents. You inhale through the canister's mouthpiece the same as you would with a breath-activated inhaler.

Dry powder inhaler

A dry powder inhaler delivers medication in the form of a powder rather than an aerosol mist. A capsule of medication as dry powder is inserted into the canister. Twisting the canister opens the capsule and releases the medicine, which you inhale through the mouthpiece.

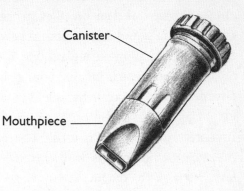

Canister

Mouthpiece

One disadvantage with powder is the amount of coordination you need to load the capsule into some inhalers. This could be a problem for young or old people or for people with arthritis, Parkinson's disease, or other neurologic disease. Depending upon your ability to breathe in deeply, you could inhale variable amounts of medication. Another concern involves the effect of humidity on dry powder, which may influence dose strength. Talk to your doctor if these factors might be problems.

NEBULIZERS

The nebulizer (see illustration on page 135) is another form of inhaler. This machine acts as a vaporizer or humidifier, delivering sprayed asthma medicine so that a person can breathe it in through a mouthpiece or face mask. Different models are available for home and hospital use. Home units are miniature versions of hospital units and can run by electricity, batteries, or automobile cigarette lighters.

Each unit works the same way. Liquid medication mixes with

water and converts, or nebulizes, into a fine spray inside the machine. The person then breathes in the spray. As more medications come in liquid form, nebulizers will allow for mixing more than one medication during a single 5- to 15-minute sitting.

Nebulizers benefit infants, young children, older people, and anyone unable to operate handheld inhalers with or without spacers. Many people find it easier to breathe regularly with a nebulizer instead of trying to inhale a deep breath and coordinate releasing medication, as with metered-dose inhalers. Nevertheless, the larger medicine doses you get from nebulizers increase the risk of side effects. Studies have shown metered-dose inhalers to be as effective as nebulizers in delivering medication to the lungs. Hospitals frequently provided medication in nebulizers to treat emergency asthma episodes, but they are now converting to metered-dose inhalers.

Oral Medication

Besides inhalers, many asthma medications are manufactured as pills or liquids that are swallowed. Oral medications benefit you by reaching into small bronchial tubes that most inhaled medication cannot reach. Newer developments in longer-acting, timed-release medicines are better at adapting to the needs and lifestyles of many individuals.

The amount of medicine people with asthma absorb over a given time period can vary. You may take five or six times longer than your neighbor to digest medication that regulates the same symptoms. That means your body requires a different dose and frequency of medication to reverse your breathing problems.

Pharmaceutical companies have responded to these variances.

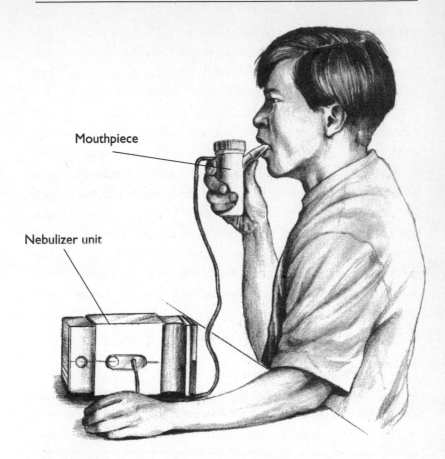

Mouthpiece

Nebulizer unit

Nebulizer

This type of inhaler is similar to a vaporizer. The nebulizer unit mixes water and medication into a fine mist or spray, which is inhaled through a mouthpiece. You do not need to coordinate inhalation with release of the medication, making nebulizers an option for people having difficulty using inhalers. Nebulizers for small children may have a mask that covers the nose and mouth instead of a mouthpiece.

Makers of medications realize children tend to balk at carrying a handheld device that may draw attention to their differences from other children, and they understand that busy people may forget midday doses. Chemists have devised tablets available by prescription that have mechanisms for releasing medication into the bloodstream at intervals throughout the day. You gain around-the-clock protection and a good night's sleep taking fewer pills.

The problem with oral medications is that the bloodstream delivers them throughout the body, not just the lungs, where they are needed. If negative or unpleasant side effects occur, they last the entire time span of the medication because the chemical is continually released into your bloodstream. Depending upon the form and dose, day-long oral medication may be more difficult for your system to balance throughout a 12- or 24-hour period.

ASTHMA MEDICATIONS: PROS AND CONS

Choosing asthma medications from among so many types can be overwhelming. Luckily, that is what your physician is trained to do. But this is your body and your asthma, and you are the person taking the medications. If you learn about your medication options, you become a partner in selecting the right medicine for you. Understanding what is available can help you control your illness and determining the kind of care you want. Begin by sorting out medication options.

Medication therapy generally follows two routes. One is to relieve symptoms quickly. The other treats airways continuously to reduce the inflammation that is always present with asthma. This prevents your asthma from recurring.

Pharmaceutical companies offer many different asthma medications under varying brand names. Most drugs can be classified according to one of these two therapy paths. The medications are known as bronchodilators (quick relief) or anti-inflammatories (long-term preventive).

Bronchodilators

Bronchodilators are medicines that act by relaxing the muscles that surround your airways, thereby opening your bronchial tubes. They relieve asthma flare-ups after they start and can help avert attacks or minimize them once they begin. The primary categories of bronchodilators are beta$_2$ agonists, methylxanthines, and anticholinergics; each is discussed in detail in this section.

Bronchodilators complement preventive medication used to treat more serious cases of asthma. Most often, bronchodilators are prescribed in an inhaler (aerosol) form, but are also available as liquid, tablets, capsules, and fluid for injection. A bronchodilator inhaler is small and easy to keep with you in case your asthma suddenly flares. It is your first line of defense when you have an attack.

Drugs that relieve acute asthma episodes go back to the early 1900s. The first oral medication to hit the asthma market was epinephrine, also called adrenaline, a hormone produced during the "fight or flight" response of the sympathetic (involuntary) nervous system. The adrenal gland produces adrenaline naturally, but researchers learned to reproduce it in the laboratory.

Epinephrine was once the first choice for treating acute asthma. But epinephrine proved a weak bronchodilator whose action fades quickly. Moreover, epinephrine has very potent effects on the heart, causing rapid heart beats, high blood pressure, nervousness, headache, and sometimes even panic attacks. People who use epinephrine develop a tolerance over time; gradually, they need more medicine to serve the same purpose. However, physicians still inject adrenaline into the bloodstream to relieve severe asthma emergencies. Be sure that only someone with special training gives you such an injection. People whose allergic reactions are very severe can receive epinephrine at home using a device called an EpiPen.

Physicians describe epinephrine as nonselective; that is, the medication acts on both the lungs and the heart. Newer, better bronchodilators that act on the lungs alone have largely replaced the routine use of epinephrine. These drugs are called beta$_2$ agonists.

BETA$_2$ AGONISTS

Beta$_2$ agonists stimulate the sympathetic nervous system, similar to adrenaline. They act on receptors located in nerve endings inside the lungs. An agonist is something that provokes; thus, beta$_2$ agonists provoke specific beta$_2$ receptors in muscles encasing the bronchial tubes to reverse. When the drug stimulates these receptors, bronchial muscles relax and bronchial tubes dilate.

Pros. Beta$_2$ agonists last longer in the body than adrenaline and result in less risk of high blood pressure or speeded heart rate. Beta$_2$ agonists are the drug family of choice for safe, short-acting medication to relax airway muscles and relieve symptoms. Beta$_2$ agonists come in every form of medication, which helps individualize treatment. Injections of beta$_2$ agonists work quickly in case of emergency, although the effect lasts only about 20 minutes. Two to four puffs of an inhaled beta$_2$ agonist taken before exercise or travel in cold air can block wheezing for up to 4 hours.

More recently, salmeterol, a longer-acting inhaled $beta_2$ agonist, has become available by prescription. Long-acting $beta_2$ agonists are taken twice a day and last up to 12 hours. Their longer action helps prevent interruptions from nighttime symptoms and lessens the number of times you must remember to use your inhaler.

Cons. Even longer-acting $beta_2$ agonists cannot control unstable asthma. While $beta_2$ agonists are considered a "rescue" medication to be used to relieve short-term symptoms, they also can be used with some patients for long-term control. Studies have failed to show that this medication may reverse chronic airway inflammation found in asthma, necessitating use of an anti-inflammatory drug to prevent symptoms.

$Beta_2$ agonists cause difficulties if taken too much and for too long. Inhaling more than one canister a month indicates an excessive reliance on bronchodilators to improve asthma. Overuse can lead to poor asthma control. Some evidence suggests that regular use of $beta_2$ agonists can decrease their potency. Many people with severe asthma prefer a $beta_2$ agonist for quicker action than anti-inflammatory medications, which take days to act. But they then expose themselves to potentially fatal or near fatal attacks from asthma that flares out of control. If you find you are inhaling short-term medication once or twice each day, contact your physician. You need to add medication to your treatment plan that prevents symptoms from occurring.

Taking a $beta_2$ agonist through an inhaler results in fewer major side effects than $beta_2$ agonist pills. But patients who inhale them report problems, too. The most common complaint is shakiness. Another noticeable side effect is a heartbeat that races or pounds. (These side effects tend to ease up over time.)

Taking a beta$_2$ agonist as a pill intensifies these side effects because more medication is absorbed into the bloodstream in pill form than with an inhaler. People taking the pills report tremors, nervousness, thumping heart, muscle cramps, and sleeplessness.

Beta$_2$ agonists and beta blockers. You may be confused about different beta receptors. As mentioned, beta$_2$ receptors are present in the lungs. But other beta receptors are located in different organs, such as the heart. These are known as beta$_1$ receptors. Medications to treat heart disease that target beta$_1$ receptors in heart tissue are called beta blockers. Beta blockers are also prescribed for abnormal swelling in the eye (glaucoma), high blood pressure, and migraine headaches.

One theory proposes that people with asthma have blocked beta receptors, a condition either inherited or acquired during illness. This means their receptors easily constrict rather than dilate airways as they should. Taking beta blockers triggers constriction, the blocking response, and asthma flare-ups as well. This

---

COMMON BETA$_2$ AGONISTS*

Albuterol (Airet, Proventil, Ventolin)
Metaproterenol (Alupent, Metaprel)
Isoetharine (Bronkometer, Bronkosol)
Salmeterol (Serevent)
Isoproterenol (Isuprel, Medihaler, Medihaler-Iso)
Terbutaline (Bricanyl, Brethaire)
Procaterol
Pirbuterol (Maxair)
Salbutamol
Bitolterol (Tornalate)

---

*Generic drug names are given first; examples of common brand names are in parentheses.

includes beta blocker eyedrops that seep into the bloodstream through the eye. Always remember to tell your eye doctor you have asthma before beginning glaucoma treatment.

METHYLXANTHINES

Before inhalers, methylxanthines were the leading asthma medications. They could be administered intravenously or by pill, tablets, or liquid. Theophylline was formerly the most widely prescribed bronchodilator in the methylxanthine category and a keystone of asthma treatment in the US. But recently, controversies over the medication's benefits and action have clouded the drug's popularity.

Exactly how theophylline works in the lungs remains unclear. Reports indicate that theophylline inhibits mast cells in the airway lining from discharging chemicals, such as histamine. It suppresses cell migration that triggers allergic asthma symptoms. Recent studies report that theophylline acts as an anti-inflammatory during the later phase of asthma episodes. Theophylline may also relax airway muscles, allowing the tubes to open and airflow to continue.

Pros. Theophylline provides short- and long-term alternatives for people who cannot tolerate beta$_2$ agonists. The drug reduces mucus buildup and blocks nighttime symptoms in mild to moderate asthmas. Its long-term benefits for preventing symptoms are well documented for up to 12 hours, although theophylline is generally less effective than beta$_2$ agonists. New studies suggest that methylxanthines may reduce swelling.

The medication comes in tablets and capsules of varying strengths and is available with a time-released formula. Caffeine is considered a methylxanthine drug, so you may want to watch

COMMON METHYLXANTHINE MEDICATIONS

Theophylline (Theo-Dur, Theolair, Slo-bid, Uniphyl, Theo-24)
Aminophylline

---

your coffee, tea, and chocolate intake when on this asthma medication.

Some people prefer taking one or two pills each day to inhaling medication several times a day. Longer-acting medications offer you the ease of remembering your medication less often. Timed-release doses provide more balanced, around-the-clock coverage. They enhance the effects of inhaled corticosteroids for nighttime protection, to help you sleep uninterrupted. Ideally, controlled-release or delayed-release pills distribute theophylline into the bloodstream continuously until your next dose.

Cons. Some of the benefits of theophylline—a delayed reaction and timed-release options—are also its drawbacks. The rate of medication released into the bloodstream varies greatly, and absorption into the bloodstream varies with the individual. What you eat, and when, has an impact on theophylline absorption. These make controlling dosages difficult. On the plus side, there are enough dose choices to suit most people with asthma. On the negative side, this may mean more trial and error to find the right option.

Another major drawback with theophylline involves the number and seriousness of side effects. Usually, the amount of medication you receive depends upon your body weight. With asthma, the severity of your symptoms compound the picture.

Too much theophylline in your body can be dangerous. The

body digests theophylline in the liver. Any malfunction in the liver slows the rate at which the body rids itself of medication. Taking other medications, such as cimetidine and certain antibiotics, and having a fever further slows the body's ability to eliminate theophylline. The result is a higher blood level of theophylline and systemwide problems as the amount of the drug in your system reaches toxic levels.

The number and seriousness of adverse effects increase with the amount of theophylline toxicity. Usually, these reactions reverse once you stop medications. Therefore, you may need to have your blood tested to monitor theophylline levels for any indication of problems.

Warning: The following symptoms of theophylline toxicity require immediate medical attention. Go to a hospital emergency department or call your physician right away if you experience any of these symptoms:

- Nausea or vomiting
- Diarrhea
- Confusion
- Seizures
- Headache
- Fluttery heartbeat

Call your physician promptly if you experience:

- Frequent sleeplessness
- Frequent urination
- Long-term intestinal problems
- Unexplained blotches on your skin that may indicate reversible liver damage (very rare)

Be cautious of giving your child theophylline. Some studies suggest that theophylline causes learning and behavior difficulties. Children who become restless or agitated as a result of the drug appear more easily distracted and prone to aggression. Although conflicting reports have surfaced since initial investigations, watch your child for clues of adverse effects from theophylline or any asthma medication. Should your physician prescribe theophylline, follow these simple guidelines:

- Do not chew theophylline in tablet or capsule form. Too much timed-release medicine will discharge at once.
- Always take theophylline with food. You will have less chance of an upset stomach.
- Never mix theophylline with hot food. The medicine will dissolve and release too much into your system at one time.
- You can open only the capsules and mix the contents with a small amount of sweet, soft foods, such as applesauce or jelly.

ANTICHOLINERGICS

Several ancient cultures understood that certain agents known as anticholinergics, found in herbal preparations, relieved breathing diseases. Blended leaves of the *Atropa belladonna* (atropine) and *Datura stramonium* (stramonium) plants calmed internal organs. People with asthma breathed easier after smoking cigarettes laced with stramonium until the late 1800s. Physicians later realized that the problems from inhaling paper and other chemicals outweighed the benefits of "asthma cigarettes."

Today, atropine and newer, more effective anticholinergics such as ipratopium bromide, continue to relieve breathing disor-

COMMON ANTICHOLINERGICS

Atropine (from the *Atropa belladonna* plant)
Ipratropium bromide (Atrovent)

ders, including asthma. When used for asthma, they are not used as the first line of defense, but rather to supplement beta$_2$ agonists. They are not primarily used for asthma alone. Anticholinergics act on different nerves than do the beta$_2$ agonists, although both block nerve pathways to the lung, altering muscle tone in the bronchial wall. Anticholinergics stimulate specific lung nervous system receptors, or cholinergics, in the vagus nerve. This nerve branches into smooth muscles responsible for airway opening and mucous glands that discharge thick secretions. The result is reduced inflammation and relaxed bronchial muscles. Throughout the respiratory tract, the drug stimulates nerve activity in other reactive cells to decrease mouth and lung secretions.

Pros. Newer drugs are better at targeting only the lungs. They show fewer side effects than do older anticholinergics, such as atropine, because less of the drug becomes absorbed into the bloodstream. Many physicians prefer anticholinergics for relief of acute bronchospasm as an alternative to beta$_2$ agonists or when prescribed to boost beta$_2$ agonist action. Research has shown that anticholinergics decrease mucous secretions and inhibit the negative effects of cholinergics. They are also used for treatment of chronic bronchitis, which is characterized by excess mucus production in the lungs.

Cons. Some people on anticholinergics notice dry mouth and throat and more wheezing. Physicians see disadvantages in that anticholinergics only relieve bronchospasm initiated by cholinergics. The medications do not treat exercise-induced asthma or allergic asthmas. Anticholinergics take longer to start working than do beta$_2$ agonists—which is the main reason that beta$_2$ agonists are the most prescribed bronchodilator drug for asthma.

Anti-inflammatory Medications

In 1991, a panel of international experts recommended a new treatment focus that identified asthma as an ongoing problem involving airway inflammation. On the basis of current research and similar studies from the mid-1980s, they offered a treatment shift away from calming acute flare-ups to preventing serious attacks. The panel's report agreed that bronchodilators work best for acute asthma situations and for preventive pretreatment before exertion or exercise. But it emphasized corticosteroid anti-inflammatory drugs as the foundation for preventive treatment for asthma.

The revised approach relies on daily medication to maintain healthy lungs. It recommends that patients who require regularly administered bronchodilators switch to longer-acting drugs designed to reduce airway swelling. Some anti-inflammatories, however, can take from days to weeks before they reduce symptoms. The length of this delay discourages many people with asthma, tempting them to stop taking their preventive medicine. The result is inadequate treatment that can lead to needless worsening of the condition. Asthma deaths have doubled since 1978, and some researchers attribute this increase to reluctance to adhere to daily medication schedules. Staying with a medication regimen boils down to tradeoffs that influence quality of life. Do the disadvantages of constantly taking medications outweigh the current and potential problems with asthma flare-ups?

There is a substantial amount of evidence from studies to suggest that patients with even mild or no obvious symptoms showed inflamed airways. This suggested that the best way to relieve symptoms was to add anti-inflammatory medications to treatment plans.

Anti-inflammatory medications operate deep inside the airways where inflammation begins. Their job is to block production of substances of cells involved in inflammation, such as mast cells. This action reduces or reverses swelling that causes asthma symptoms. Equally important, these medications lessen airway sensitivity. This prevents swelling from occurring, which keeps airways open. If your asthma symptoms appear more than once or twice a week and less powerful options cannot control them, your physician will probably prescribe an anti-inflammatory medication.

Before newer drugs were developed, the only anti-inflammatory drug was a corticosteroid pill, such as prednisone. Oral corticosteroids caused plenty of serious side effects, giving the entire drug family a bad reputation. Now several types of anti-inflammatory drugs come in inhaled form, greatly reducing negative reactions. The four primary types of anti-inflammatories are corticosteroids (steroids), mast cell stabilizers (nonsteroids), antiallergic drugs, and antileukotriene drugs.

ORAL CORTICOSTEROIDS

The most common group of anti-inflammatories are oral corticosteroids (steroids). Reports about side effects from oral or injected doses may scare some people with asthma. Yet oral or intravenous

COMMON ORAL CORTICOSTEROIDS

Betamethasone (Celestone)
Dexamethasone (Decadron)
Prednisone (Deltasone)
Cortisone (Cortone)
Hydrocortisone (Hydrocortone)
Methylprednisolone (Medrol)

corticosteroids can be a miraculous last resort for severe uncontrolled asthma or acute attacks.

The medication you take is actually a synthetic version of the natural steroids produced in your adrenal glands. These triangle-shaped glands sit on top of the kidneys and give off hormones that affect several important functions, including:

- Regulating body salts, which balances sodium and potassium and fluid retention
- Reducing inflammation, the action that helps control asthma symptoms
- Serving as a weak male hormone in males and females
- Helping the body metabolize carbohydrates, fats, and proteins
- Releasing added steroids as protection from physical stress
- Helping control heart rate and blood pressure

Corticosteroids prescribed for asthma are very different from the steroids you might hear that some athletes misuse. Athletes take steroids that mimic hormones produced in male testicles to strengthen muscles. Corticosteroids used in the treatment of asthma are adrenal hormones.

When you take corticosteroids for your asthma, the medication becomes absorbed into the bloodstream and travels throughout your system until it reaches the lungs. Once in the lungs, corticosteroids prevent cells from causing airway swelling. Exposing your body to significant amounts of corticosteroids for prolonged periods can affect other organ systems such as your bones and skin. For this reason, oral and injected corticosteroids are tightly controlled. Your physician will monitor your airflow with spirometry or peak flow to determine whether oral corticosteroids are necessary and at what dose.

If you have severe asthma, your doses will probably be higher for longer periods of time. They may be tapered off over a period of 1 to 3 weeks. Usually, corticosteroids are taken when you awaken, which mimics the body's natural steroid production schedule. If you have nighttime symptoms, your doctor may split your dose between morning and night. Some physicians recommend taking oral corticosteroids on alternating days. They contend this gives the adrenal gland time to adjust, producing fewer side effects.

Pros. Oral corticosteroids are powerful anti-inflammatory medications. They are easy to administer and offer fast, dramatic reversal of symptoms during life-threatening asthma situations. Even though some corticosteroids take a few hours to work, their protection lasts longer. Oral corticosteroids can be used for a brief period to gain control of asthma before moving to other long-term treatments with fewer side effects.

Cons. A disadvantage of oral corticosteroids is the array of negative side effects associated with taking large doses of the drug over long periods of time. Because the corticosteroids enter the bloodstream and travel throughout the body, there is potential for damage to other organs. This should not stop you from taking corticosteroids, though, if your physician recommends them for severe asthma. Taking corticosteroids just means you need to be more diligent about identifying and reporting any side effects.

The adrenal glands rely on the extra steroids and stop producing natural ones. Eventually, the adrenal glands shut down from disuse. When medication ends, the adrenal glands remain nonfunctional. Usually, they begin producing steroids again after a while. Until they energize, however, the body may experience steroid withdrawal symptoms from the discontinued supply of steroids. You may feel weak, tired, achy, or feverish. Suddenly stopping your corticosteroids after you have been taking them for a long time can potentially be fatal. Therefore, it is unwise to suddenly stop oral corticosteroids without your physician's knowledge. Other potential side effects from long-term use of oral corticosteroids include the following:

- Weak bones (osteoporosis)
- Retarded growth in young children
- Cataracts
- Fluid retention
- Muscle weakness
- Increased appetite and accompanying weight gain
- High blood pressure
- Increased blood sugar levels
- Altered skin (thinning, acne, easily bruised, rash)
- Headache, seizures
- Risk of stomach ulcers
- Unwanted hair growth

- Increased risk of infection
- Mood swings

INHALED CORTICOSTEROIDS

Inhaled corticosteroids offer a major advance in asthma treatment. Because they are inhaled straight into the airways, much less is absorbed into your system. Instead, they concentrate on reducing swelling in the airways and improving results obtained from bronchodilators.

Your doctor may prescribe a beta$_2$ agonist with an inhaled corticosteroid. The beta$_2$ agonist is puffed first to unblock airways so the corticosteroid can penetrate deeper.

Pros. Inhaled corticosteroids help treat severe asthma with much fewer side effects than those from oral corticosteroids. Newer versions come in nebulizer and dry powder forms, which are propellant free. Use of inhaled corticosteroids for 1 month or longer significantly decreases airway inflammation. Research has shown that the drug improves breathing, decreases airway sensitivity, and results in fewer symptoms and severe episodes. Once asthma stabilizes, inhaled corticosteroids ultimately reduce the need for oral corticosteriods. One study compared treatments with inhaled corticosteroids and other medications. The results showed that people who used inhaled corticosteroids were half as likely to be hospitalized. The lowest hospitalization rates were seen in those people with asthma who combined inhaled corticosteroids with beta$_2$ agonists.

Cons. People who take inhaled corticosteroids complain about the lack of immediate symptom relief and cite it as a major reason for not taking the medicine. Although risks of serious corticosteroid problems are greatly reduced with inhalers, they do

COMMON INHALED CORTICOSTEROIDS

Beclomethasone dipropionate (Beclovent, Becloforte, Vanceril)
Dexamethasone (Decadron Phosphate, Dexacort Phosphate)
Flunisolide (AeroBid, Bronalide)
Triamcinolone acetonide (Azmacort)
Budesonide (available in dry powder inhaler)

exist. Prolonged use of high doses can increase your chances for the same types of unpleasant symptoms attributed to the pill form—although the doses of the inhaled corticosteroid would have to be very high to have a risk of side effects equal to that from oral corticosteroids. Ask your physician to provide you with the lowest dose that controls your asthma and to plan for further reduction.

Two known adverse reactions are throat irritation or thrush (candidiasis), a yeast infection in the mouth and back of the throat. Thrush can develop if you are taking an antibiotic at the same time as the corticosteroid inhaler or if you have other health problems, such as diabetes. You know you have thrush if your mouth feels gummy inside and you notice whitish patches on the back of your throat. The infection may or may not cause sore throat as well.

Call your physician if you have suspicious symptoms. A reduction in medication may alleviate the problem, or you may need to gargle with nystatin mouthwash. Either course should eliminate the thrush within a week.

To prevent thrush, rinse your mouth after each inhaler treatment. Gargle with warm water to remove any medication left in your throat. Be sure to use a spacer when inhaling corticosteroids. Spacers deliver medicine particles into the lung, rather than to the mouth and throat, where they can contribute to the development of thrush.

MAST CELL STABILIZERS

Mast cell stabilizers are long-term medications that reduce symptoms of early and delayed stages of asthma flare-ups. How they work is still unclear. They appear to stabilize mast cells in the airways, blocking them from releasing powerful chemicals, such as histamines and eosinophils, into nearby tissues and causing inflammation.

Mast cell stabilizers offer great hope for new and improved medications. Entire classes of anti-inflammatory drugs are being developed from research into the many chemicals released from mast cells.

Pros. Mast cell stabilizers have few side effects and are considered the safest family of asthma medications. Cromolyn sodium, the most common mast cell stabilizer, is derived from khellin, an Egyptian herbal treatment. Mast cell stabilizers are effective preventive medications that can substitute for corticosteroids and theophylline, especially if your asthma is mild, yet persistent. Physicians frequently choose these drugs to control mild to moderate asthma.

These drugs are particularly useful in treating children. Childhood asthma seems to be more closely related to allergies and thus seems to respond well to these nonsteroidal anti-inflammatory drugs (NSAIDs). They may also work in some adults with asthma. If taken 30 minutes before exertion or exercise, they can be useful in preventing exercise-induced asthma.

COMMON MAST CELL STABILIZERS

Cromolyn sodium (Intal)
Nedocromil sodium (Tilade)
Ketotifen

When taken regularly, mast cell stabilizers prevent airway linings from swelling in reaction to cold air, allergens, and the irritant sulfur diozide. NSAIDs come in metered-dose, powder inhaler, and nebulizer forms.

Cons. While mast cell stabilizers can prevent some asthmas, they offer limited relief once an attack starts. To maintain potency throughout the day, they must be taken four times a day, which can prove cumbersome. In addition, cromolyn sodium is slow acting. You may need to take the medication for 3 to 6 weeks before you notice improvement.

Some people experience minor side effects—a dry cough, throat irritation, skin hives, and, less often nausea. The biggest complaint, however, is that the drug leaves an undesirable aftertaste. Although uncomfortable, these complaints are minimal compared with the risks from theophylline and corticosteroids.

ANTIALLERGIC DRUGS
Similar to mast cell inhibitors, the concept of antiallergic medications as a separate category is under intense study. The idea behind antiallergic drugs is simple—eliminate the allergic reaction, and allergic asthma symptoms are greatly reduced. Exactly how antiallergic drugs act is unclear. However, research suggests that

---

COMMON ANTIALLERGICS

APPROVED IN THE US

Ketotifen

APPROVED OUTSIDE THE US

Amlexanox, azelastine, ibudilast, ozagrel, pemirolast, repinast, tazanolast, tranilast

---

these medications inhibit either mast cell activity generally or mast cell mediator release in particular.

Pros. Most studies of oral antiallergic drugs indicate that these drugs succeed in offering some improvement of mild to moderate asthma symptoms, resulting in the need for less medication of other kinds. Patients' results improved after 2 months of treatment and were most significant for children and young adults.

Cons. Antiallergic drugs focus on only one type of asthma trigger—allergies. They do not replace inhaler medications. These drugs can cause drowsiness, especially in adults during the first weeks of treatment. A common anti-allergic drug, ketotifen, may also prompt weight gain. Many antiallergics are only available in countries outside the US. Another concern is that they are available only in pill form, which magnifies adverse effects.

ANTILEUKOTRIENE MEDICATIONS

Antileukotriene medications, the first of which were released in late 1996, are the first new class of asthma medications released in decades. Leukotrienes are chemical messengers produced by

COMMON ANTILEUKOTRIENE MEDICATIONS

APPROVED IN THE US

Montelukast (Singulair)
Zafirlukast (Accolate)
Zileuton (Zyflo)

APPROVED OUTSIDE THE US

Pranlukast (Ultair)

inflammatory cells. These chemicals allow inflammatory cells to communicate with each other. There are two types of antileukotriene drugs: (1) leukotriene synthesis inhibitors, which prevent these chemicals from being generated, and (2) leukotriene receptor antagonists, which prevent these chemicals from delivering their messages by blocking their receptors.

Pros. Antileukotriene drugs are strong and very effective in preventing asthma caused by exercise. They can also prevent the development of bronchospasm caused by aspirin and may be useful in milder forms of asthma. Their role in moderate to severe asthma is currently being investigated.

Cons. Antileukotriene drugs may be effective in some people with asthma. At present, however, there is no way to predict whether a person with asthma will experience an improvement with any of these agents. A trial therapy is the only way to tell if the drugs will work in your case. Antileukotrienes produce more serious side effects than do other anti-inflammatory drugs. Reversible liver problems, headache, and nausea are some of the reported drawbacks. Physicians caution pregnant women against taking these drugs, but not earlier NSAIDs. If you take antileukotrienes, be sure to check your blood levels for the drug regularly. This way, your physician can monitor for potential liver problems.

The Search for New Medications

As long as risks exist from asthma medications, research will continue for new and improved medications. Right now, many new medications are being tested for their ability to relieve and prevent asthma. The goal for many people is to find a healthier alternative for oral corticosteroids.

If you are asked to participate in studies involving experimental drugs, weigh your decision carefully. Learn as much as you can about the drug and its side effects. Make medication choices based on your quality of life now and what could happen while taking new medicines. Medications' side effects differ but could range from nausea, headache, and stomach pain on the mild side to liver damage, worsening asthma, heart disease, and seizures at the extreme. Do these risks outweigh the benefits of eliminating corticosteroids from your treatment plan?

Other Medications

Allergies, colds, and flu can make you feel terrible. Before you discovered that you had asthma, you relieved the discomforts of ordinary illness with over-the-counter medications. You may think they would help with asthma symptoms, also. But now you are on one, two, maybe three different asthma medications. **Warning: Be cautious about taking any over-the-counter drugs**

in combination with your asthma medicine. Consult with your physician first.

ANTIHISTAMINES

This family of medications blocks the effects of histamine, the chemical released during an allergic reaction. They are available in both prescription and nonprescription forms. Antihistamines control itching, redness, and swelling in tissues throughout the body, such as skin, eyes, and nose. Although many people presume they reduce swelling in the lungs as well, this is not necessarily true.

Earlier antihistamines often made asthma worse. The drying that reduced tissue swelling resulted in thicker mucous plugging and, in some cases, airway narrowing. Most antihistamines caused sleepiness, which made continuing normal activities difficult.

Newer prescription nondrowsy antihistamines may be unpredictable in their effects when asthma is present. Some people experience no worsening of their asthma and possibly slight improvement. Other people with asthma remain sensitive to the slightest medication changes and should always be cautious. The body may build resistance to an antihistamine over time, requiring a change in medication or dose.

Watch for label warnings about asthma complications on any medication you buy. Consult your physician before taking antihistamines if you are:

- Allergic to any medication
- Pregnant or intend to become pregnant while on asthma medication

- Breast-feeding
- Taking other prescription medication

or if you have any of the following:

- Other chronic medical illnesses, such as hypertension (high blood pressure), diabetes or hypoglycemia (too much or too little sugar in the blood), or thyroid problems (overactive or underactive)
- Glaucoma
- Enlarged prostate

DECONGESTANTS

Medications that are decongestants reduce nasal congestion by narrowing blood vessels in membranes lining the nose. The results are decreased swelling, inflammation, and mucus production in nasal passages. Decongestants are found in over-the-counter cold remedies in pill, liquid, nose drop, or spray forms. Besides being used to treat colds, they are frequently recommended to relieve symptoms of hay fever and other allergies. Pseudoephedrine, phenylpropanolamine, and phenylephrine are three common decongestants available without prescription.

Decongestants can produce side effects of nervousness, nausea, and headache. These side effects increase when compounded with asthma medications that can also produce these unwanted symptoms. They are usually not recommended for people who have heart problems or prostate problems and should be carefully monitored with other asthma medication. Attempting to discontinue nose drops or sprays after lengthy use can cause a "rebound" effect, in which congestion reappears or worsens. With most drops, medication overdose causes an opposite reaction from the drug's intended use.

MUCOLYTICS AND EXPECTORANTS

Mucolytics are prescription drugs that destroy or dissolve mucus buildup in airways. Expectorants, often nonprescription, help thin and loosen mucus. With thinner mucus, coughing and clearing the airways become easier. Physicians disagree, however, about the value of mucolytics and expectorants for people with asthma.

Different medications produce a wide range of reactions. For example, acetylcysteine, a prescription mucolytic, irritates asthmatic airways, emits a sulfurlike smell, and can cause gagging, nausea, and vomiting. Iodides may produce a bronchodilator reaction, and they are suitable for only short-term treatment. After longer durations, they can cause increased salivation, skin eruptions, and thyroid disease. These are rarely recommended for children and pregnant women.

Guaifenesin, an expectorant, is found in many nonprescription cough medicines, but it has little value. Guaifenesin usually works to increase lung fluid production that helps thin mucus, although some people find it irritates their airways. Some guaifenesin preparations are available only by prescription.

Water is a good expectorant. Many people find relief by drinking large amounts of fluids during an asthma attack. Others advocate inhaling steam to relieve bronchial congestion. Some physicians are not convinced that water actually helps thin mucus. Nonprescription aerosols with water may make asthma worse, but this may be a function of the chemical propellant rather than the sprayed water. Salt water produces inconsistent reactions. Still, drinking about six glasses of water a day is important for keeping your entire body functioning better.

ANTIBIOTICS

Antibiotics are useful in clearing up bacteria from the respiratory system. Most infections, however, are viral, and antibiotics cannot cure symptoms from viral infections. Thus, antibiotics have no place in the routine treatment of asthma. Antibiotics never get rid of the common asthma triggers or contribute to shorter hospital stays after severe attacks.

GASTRIC REFLUX

The first line of defense with gastric reflux is prevention. To relieve the backup of stomach acid that triggers your asthma, follow the measures suggested in Chapter 4. Should these recommendations fail to prevent gastric reflux, your physician may prescribe antacid medications. Popular prescription medications that reduce acid backup include cisapride, omeprazole, and ranitidine. Many nonprescription drugs are available, too; talk to your physician.

Very severe gastric reflux in some people may not improve with high doses of medication and may require surgery. The goal of surgery is to strengthen the esophageal sphincter, the one-way valve between esophagus and stomach, to stop reflux. This surgery is not always successful. Have your doctor make sure your reflux really causes the asthma before you agree to surgery.

DAY-TO-DAY LIFE WITH ASTHMA MEDICATION

If you are like many people with asthma, you rely on medication to breathe better. Prescribing medications is your physician's job. But blending medicines into your daily schedule and following their progress is up to you. The National Institutes of Health (NIH) offers these hints to help you follow your prescribed guidelines:

- Take medication at the same time each day. Integrate taking medicine into your regular routines. For example, use your inhaler at mealtime, before brushing your teeth, or as part of bedtime activities.
- Remind yourself to take medications by putting a note on the refrigerator, calendar, or bathroom mirror. Set a timer or alarm clock, or wear something in a different way, such as a ring on a different finger, to help you remember your medication.
- Involve family members in helping you remember. Ask someone to remind you about your medication schedule.

SAMPLE MEDICATION CHECKLIST

NAME	DATES (FROM–TO)	STRENGTH	RESULTS/ADVERSE EFFECTS
Salmeterol	10/96–11/97	Metered dose	Coughing; bitter taste
Albuterol	12/96	Metered dose	Works better; tastes good
Cromolyn Sodium	1/97	Metered dose	So far so good; pain to remember 4 × /day

- Carry a beta₂ agonist inhaler with you at all times. You never know when an asthma emergency will strike.

- Order an extra inhaler, so you have one to carry with you and one to keep at home, work, or school. Having a backup inhaler makes good sense.

- Keep track of the medications you take. Prepare a checklist to help you. The medication checklist on page 162 is a sample.

MEDICATION PRECAUTIONS

Medications can lose their effectiveness. To achieve maximum results from your medicines, follow these guidelines:

- **Watch dates on medication labels.** Labels tell you when your medication will expire and lose potency or when the propellant will lose its strength. Some medicines actually spoil if they lay around too long.

- **Do not take medicine in the dark.** The chance of taking the wrong medicine is too great.

- **Throw away any medicine that is outdated and prescription drugs you no longer need.** Before your asthma is under control, you may go through several medications that remain unfinished. Get rid of them, too. Asthma medicine is strong. You do not want anyone, including yourself, taking something by accident at a later date.

- **Keep all medication out of your children's reach.** Your children may be curious about the containers you put inside your mouth each day. If your child has asthma, be a good role model—keep medications in a safe place and teach your child a cautious respect for all medicines. If you have small children, call the local

Poison Control Center for stickers with easy-to-understand pictures on them, such as "Mr. Yuk," that indicate something is poisonous. Scary cartoon characters help boys and girls learn that canisters and bottles of asthma medication are off limits.

- **Store medications away from heat and direct light.** Do not store bronchodilators in the bathroom medicine chest. Bathroom heat and humidity can cause medication to break down and lose its strength.

- **Make sure liquid medicines do not freeze.** Freezing and thawing again changes the medicine's chemical makeup and its effectiveness for your asthma.

Follow Your Treatment Plan

Constantly taking medicine can be challenging—and tedious. It can be inconvenient, costly, embarrassing, and sometimes uncomfortable. But the alternative can be much worse—even deadly. You can lessen the disruptive impact of medication by learning to accept this chronic disease. When following your medication plan:

- Stick to the medications prescribed by your physician only. Some over-the-counter drugs may react with your asthma medication. Other medications may trigger breathing or different allergic problems. Nonprescription medicines only provide temporary relief, masking the underlying problem.

- Adhere to suggested doses. In some cases, you may have to keep taking the drug for at least a couple of weeks to give the medicine a chance to act on your symptoms. Changing dose amounts makes it difficult to decide if you need more or less of a prescription. Of course, if you have adverse reactions from a drug, contact your physician immediately.

Medication Alert

If your treatment includes regular asthma medicines, particularly oral corticosteroids, you may want to wear a medical-alert bracelet or necklace. These identify you as a person with asthma who needs certain medicines. This information may be critical for health-care providers attempting to save your life during a medical emergency.

Monitor Your Medications

An important part of treatment is identifying a way to monitor medication for adverse effects. Before beginning each new medication, your physician will most likely:

- Check, or recheck, your vital signs and symptoms
- Measure your pulmonary function
- Ask about daily activities and how you are breathing
- Review what other medications you are taking and whether they work

Then it is your turn to assert your role in the patient–physician partnership. Do not leave the doctor's office with a new prescription without discussing everything you need to know about your medications. If you are using an inhaler, ask you doctor to show you how it is used. Make sure your physician writes any directions in your log or on a form like this one that you can keep with other asthma material for referral. Identify the following:

Name of medication: _____

Results you can expect from the medication: _____

Explanation of how the medicine works and when you will feel it working:

Exact dose and how to administer the medicine for what length of time (ask whether medication should be taken with food or at certain times of the day for the greatest effectiveness): _____

Reactions to expect, including positive and negative:

What to do if there are adverse reactions:

Interactions with other medicine or foods to avoid (can you drink alcoholic beverages?):

What to do if you miss a dose: _____

Availability of a less expensive generic form (if so, what is it?): _____

When should the physician be called (includes emergencies and reporting when the medication is not working): _____

NONPRESCRIPTION AND ALTERNATIVE ASTHMA TREATMENTS

Learning to live with asthma means more than mere compliance with medication schedules. Your treatment process will be more complete if you investigate all the therapeutic alternatives available to you. The more you learn about asthma, the more you will be able to:

- Help yourself feel better
- Make informed choices
- Determine your or your child's needs, which may change as the illness and new preferred treatments change
- Act as advocate for your and your child's best interests

As the number of asthma cases steadily grows, information about asthma has become more accessible. The unresolved mysteries of asthma attract considerable interest, research, and treatments. This creates more information to sort through to confirm the right approach for you.

As you search for information, you may hear about programs alleging great benefits. Some treatments may work on isolated symptoms or enhance general health. Others may be quite controversial. Be cautious about any treatment that claims a *complete cure*.

Here are some factors to consider before committing to any nonmedication treatment plan:

- Remember that the only scientifically tested treatments for asthma involve preventing asthma triggers and taking prescribed medications that work on your particular asthma symptoms. Alternative treatments can be beneficial to your overall health but not have a great deal of effect on your asthma. However, improving your overall mental and physical health may be the best insurance against a wide range of diseases, including asthma. Staying healthy and centered certainly cannot hurt!

- Be wary of treatments that claim to be "natural." Like the term *light* in food packaging, *natural* can mean almost anything. Several natural approaches, such as breathing exercises and relaxing techniques, have proven helpful in treating asthma, but other approaches involving herbs require you to take substances that are "natural" but also potentially lethal in high doses.

• Work with trained professionals only. Find out if performing certain nonmedical treatments requires licensing in your state and check whether your treatment provider has them. Talk to your physician as a point of reference.

• Investigate program claims before agreeing to follow a given plan, especially if those claims seem unrealistic. Ask the following questions:

- What is involved in treatment?
- Can treatment harm me or my asthmatic child?
- Is the approach logical and based on results proved in studies?
- What does treatment mean for my family?
- Have I been properly evaluated for this treatment?
- Does this program appear to address my individual needs, or are all participants following the same plan?
- How will progress be monitored?
- Will treatment be costly and hook our family into many months of sessions?

• Weigh the options before totally embarking on anything that interrupts a treatment plan that may be preventing your asthma attacks. Do not stop taking medication that is controlling your asthma while you search for an alternative.

• Discuss options with an objective professional or someone who understands asthma but has nothing to gain or lose by your treatment choice.

• Try to leave emotion out of your decision. Months of searching for the right medication may leave you believing you are running out of choices. When you feel uncomfortable, you may try anything to relieve the discomfort. A new alternative may seem like your last hope.

A range of alternative practices that are not part of mainstream medicine are used by alternative practitioners to treat asthma. A few have been studied scientifically under controlled conditions, but for most, little scientific research exists.

Homeopathy

Homeopathy is a system of medicine invented in the late 1700s by Samuel Hahnemann, a German physician and naturopath. Homeopathic "remedies" are natural substances, such as herbs and minerals, that have gone through a process of extreme dilution; in many remedies, the original substance can no longer be detected. At full strength, the substances are said to cause the symptoms (not the illness) being treated. According to homeopathic theory, the infinitesimal amount of the substance left after the dilution process evokes the healing power of the person's "vital force." This force is believed to be a healing energy, essentially spiritual in nature, that is present in every organism.

In homeopathy, the focus is on curing the underlying disease rather than treating symptoms, as doctors often do with medications. During initial visits, homeopaths spend a great deal of time gathering health histories from patients to identify overall well-being, symptoms, and disease patterns. They ask varied questions to ferret out clues unique to that person. Consequently, two people with asthma may receive different remedy plans.

Homeopaths believe traditional medications merely suppress

symptoms, interfering with the body's normal ability to heal itself. In homeopathy, symptoms are viewed as the body's healthy attempt to achieve balance. In theory, the infinitesimal doses of symptom-causing substances in homeopathic remedies stimulate the body's "vital force" to respond in a way that somewhat resembles an immune system reaction. New symptoms are a sign either that you need a different remedy or that your body is trying to right itself.

There are no scientifically controlled studies to suggest that homeopathy is a useful treatment for asthma. Even homeopathic practitioners report that chances for complete cures for everyone with asthma are limited. If you experience severe flare-ups, you should still continue to take your asthma medicine.

If you are interested in pursuing a course of homeopathic treatment, check the Resources section at the back of this book for referral sources. Some homeopaths are also physicians, and some homeopaths will coordinate treatment with a traditional physician. Watch out for homeopathic remedies dispensed by untrained practitioners who call themselves homeopaths. Always ask about credentials before making an appointment.

Chiropractic

Chiropractic involves treating disease by manipulating and adjusting the spinal column and other parts of the muscle and skeletal systems. The practice was first developed by Iowan Daniel Palmer in 1895. Palmer believed that a poorly aligned spine presses on nerves, causing direct pain or referred symptoms in other areas of the body. He coined the term *chiropractic* from Greek words meaning "done by hand."

Chiropractic is based on the idea that spinal misalignments of the vertebrae, or subluxations in chiropractic terminology, interfere with normal nerve transmission from the brain to the rest of the body and that this interference causes disease. Chiropractic adjustments are aimed at removing subluxations and restoring normal nerve function, which, in theory, allows the body to heal itself.

Chiropractors, like homeopaths, see their healing practices as holistic; that is, they try to treat the whole person rather than a body system or set of symptoms. The also try to use natural techniques or substances, rather than surgery or drugs. They adjust vertebrae, bones, and muscles with manipulations that can be uncomfortable initially. Chiropractic manipulation has been proven an effective treatment for common low-back pain (not arising from a herniated vertebral disc). Chiropractors claim that their therapy is effective for a wide range of ailments, including headaches and asthma. No scientific studies, however, have documented any positive effects on asthma symptoms from chiropractic manipulation.

Chiropractors are licensed in all 50 states. They must complete a 5-year course of study at an approved chiropractic college. Many physicians have working relationships with chiropractors and can refer you to one. Chiropractors are not allowed to write prescriptions for medication; thus, you will need to continue seeing your physician for asthma medication.

Acupuncture

According to Chinese medicine, a universal life force known as chi flows like a river through 12 main pathways, or meridians, which circulate through the major organs, delivering chi and giving life. As they travel, they irrigate and nourish the tissues. Good health is defined as the free flow of chi. An imbalance of chi or a blocked pathway results in ill health, much as a dam backs up a river's flow.

Acupuncturists seek to unblock obstructions and correct imbalances of chi in order to revitalize health. To do this, they insert very thin needles at specified points (acupuncture points) along the meridians. Pathways may lead far from where the affected organ lies, and acupuncturists may place needles in many spots on the body, including the face.

How acupuncture works is difficult to explain in terms of conventional science, for the simple reason that chi is not physical and is thus not measurable. Some physicians believe that insertion of the needles stimulates release of endorphins and other powerful nervous system chemicals. These block nerve endings from sending painful messages to the brain, which makes you unable to feel pain. Critics believe the positive results from acupuncture come from a placebo effect; that is, that the mind wishes the treatment would work, and so it does.

Acupuncturists decide where to place the needles by carefully taking the pulse in three different positions on both wrists. The quality or feel of the pulse signifies different types of chi imbalance. The degree of impairment affects needle temperature, angle, and depth into the skin. Some needles barely prick the skin, while others can sink an inch. Sometimes, the acupuncturist will twist or vibrate the needles. Newer variants of acupuncture involve passing a mild electrical current through the needles.

Initially, pain varies from mild to a sharp pinch. Needles stay in place for several minutes. During that time, the needle sites can tingle or feel numb or sore. On rare occasions, a small drop of blood may appear at the pinprick site.

Acupuncture is widely practiced in China, where the process began, and is gaining increasing acceptance in the west. In the US, the main focus of acupuncture treatment is in relief from chronic pain. Despite its widespread use, however, there are relatively few scientific studies that are large enough or produce definitive enough results to provide a basis upon which conventional scientists and physicians can draw conclusions.

Although a few studies on acupuncture treatment for asthma showed a modest temporary effect, the evidence is decidedly mixed. Most studies suggest that acupuncture is not effective for establishing and maintaining control over asthma. The method in which acupuncture is administered makes it an impractical choice for treatment of acute attacks.

If acupuncture interests you:

• **Find a qualified licensed practitioner.** Licensing requirements vary with each state. Some states do not require any license to practice acupuncture; in others, only physicians or dentists are allowed to practice acupuncture. In some states, licensed acupuncturists can see only those patients referred to them by physicians. Contact the American Academy of Medical Acupuncture or other agencies listed in the Resources section at the back of this book for referrals. To receive academy accreditation, physicians complete at least 200 hours of training in medical acupuncture.

• **Consult with your asthma physician.** Make sure you follow your regular treatment plan while undergoing acupuncture.

• **Check with your insurance carrier for coverage.** Some

companies cover acupuncture only when it is prescribed by a conventional physician.

- **If you are planning to donate blood, wait to begin acupuncture treatment.** Many laboratories require a 1-year waiting period from the time you last had acupuncture. This is a precaution to avoid the chance of needles' contaminating your blood.

- **Enhance treatment by following certain guidelines before you go:**

  - Request disposable needles to avoid the risk of infection.
  - Refrain from strenuous exercise, sexual activity, and alcoholic beverages at least 6 hours prior to treatment.
  - Eat only small meals before and after treatment.
  - Plan restful activities after treatment.

- **Document in writing any effects of acupuncture.** Note effects—positive and negative—so follow-up visits can be tailored to your progress.

Relaxation and Meditation

Emotions cannot cause asthma, but can make attacks worse. Psychological factors may play a role in everyday stresses that contribute to the disease. Therefore, traditional physicians as well as nontraditional practitioners often recommend techniques to reduce stress and to better deal with emotions.

Special relaxation techniques are helpful in reducing high blood pressure, stress from work or home, and pain during childbirth. For people with asthma, lowering stress alleviates the strain on lungs. Several relaxation techniques have found their roots in traditional and alternative therapy circles.

BREATHING EXERCISES

Many people with asthma fear for their next breath. When your breathing becomes impaired, pulse and blood pressure rates rise and the heart works harder. These stresses cause muscles to tense. Breathing and muscle-tensing exercises, as shown on this page and the next, can help relieve the strain.

Slow, deep, rhythmic breathing contributes to a relaxed body. A slow breathing rate increases the volume of air exchanged with each breath, decreasing the amount of air trapped in your lungs behind the narrowed bronchial passages. The balance of blood gases improves, enriching tissues throughout the system. Your lungs become better able to cough and clear. In addition, deep breathing reduces the effort of moving air in and out of airways. As your body works less to gain the air it needs, you can relax. (See "Deep Breathing Exercise" on the next page.)

Deep abdominal breathing is a more efficient exchange of air than breathing with chest muscles. For people with asthma,

---

ACTIVE RELAXATION EXERCISE

- Lie flat on the floor or sit straight up in a chair.
- Tense your right toe muscles for 5 seconds. Think about keeping the muscles tight and monitor the sensation of the muscle contraction.
- Relax your toe muscles and rest for 15 seconds.
- Repeat the tensing and releasing for each muscle group in your body. Concentrate on moving up from your toes to your forehead. Notice how you gain control over each set of muscles, particularly your lungs.
- Tense all muscles in your body.
- Release all muscles in your body.
- Practice this exercise twice a day.

BREATHING FOR RELAXATION EXERCISE

- Sit with your back straight and lean forward.
- Lay your arms flat on your upper leg, so your shoulders droop.
- Purse your lips in a whistle position.
- Breathe in through your nose slowly.
- Hold your breath for about 5 seconds.
- Breathe out slowly through your mouth.

DEEP BREATHING EXERCISE

- Stand straight or sit straight up with one hand on your abdomen and one hand lying on your chest.
- Inhale deeply through your nose.
- Feel your abdomen move in and chest expand as you take in air.
- Hold your breath for 5 seconds.
- Exhale slowly through your mouth until you are out of air.
- Feel your abdominal muscles contract to push air from the lungs.
- Practice deep breathing 5 to 10 times at least twice a day.

breathing with greater efficiency means less work for the strained respiratory muscles. More air enters the lungs with each breath. Air comes through the nose, where cilia-lined nasal passages are better equipped than the mouth to clean air going into the lungs.

Relaxing is often a matter of mind over body. If you can clear your head of the worries of the day, your muscles should relax. Several techniques help clear your mind and may ease troubled breathing.

PASSIVE RELAXATION AND MUSIC

With passive relaxation, the body remains inactive and the mind does all the work. First, find a restful position in which you can sit or lie still. Focus on a single phrase or sound to push any stresses out of your mind. As you concentrate, your muscles relax. Relaxing allows you to breathe easier.

Music can help you to achieve passive relaxation. For people who have trouble staying still long enough to relax, music gives them purpose. Studies have produced differing conclusions about the value of music in treating asthma, but most findings suggest that listening to certain music lowers muscle tension and slows breathing. The brain tends to focus on peaceful sounds—for example, ocean waves or harp music—and stimulates an array of calming body reactions. In particular, blood flow and metabolism slow. These lead to a slowdown of the breathing process, which deepens breathing with less effort.

MEDITATION

Passive relaxation is a vehicle for meditation. In meditation, you focus on a single word or object as a means of reaching a relaxed and focused mental state. As your mind drifts, you refocus your attention. Many forms of meditation use concentration on breath as the point of focus. By diligently concentrating on keeping your attention focused, you eventually free your mind of many of the distracting thoughts that fill it most of the time. This meditative state calms both the body and mind.

Studies show that meditation is a valuable tool for promoting relaxation by reducing stress, which can make asthma symptoms worse. As far back as 1962, Japanese neurophysiologists found that meditation:

- Enhances slower, more rhythmic deep breathing
- Decreases muscle tension
- Reduces pulse rate
- Lowers blood pressure

VISUALIZATION

Visualization is a relaxation technique very similar to meditation. Instead of concentrating on a single word or object, you create a mental picture of health. It helps to make the picture as vivid and as realistic as possible. You might imagine relaxed bronchial tubes and a clear and free exchange of air in the lungs. By imagining your body in a relaxed, balanced, and healthy state, you are essentially sending it a message that it is strong and can heal itself without trauma.

In theory, by creating images of health while in a relaxed state, you can change your perceptions and expectations of your disease. These changed perceptions seem to have an impact on how the immune system responds to disease, although the connection between the mind and the body is not yet fully understood.

People who regularly practice visualization report the technique helps them maintain their sense of calm and well-being. If an asthma attack occurs, visualization may be able to reduce the panic that can heighten asthma symptoms. However, if your symptoms currently are not well controlled, visualization may not be appropriate for you.

Finding calm through creating mental pictures takes practice. Books and workshops at community centers can help you learn visualization. You may benefit from trained leaders and the positive atmosphere of other participants concentrating together, which encourages your efforts to visualize. See "An Asthma Visualization" on page 180 for a visualization "script" that you might follow.

BIOFEEDBACK

Biofeedback teaches you to be aware of your body's automatic and unconscious processes, such as your skin temperature and heart rate, so that you can have some conscious control of them. In biofeedback training, you are connected to a monitoring device that records a specific body function. The machine relays information about your body's responses back to you as sounds, numbers on a screen, or other visual cues. Gradually, your mind learns to connect with how you feel when body functions change. Therapists often link biofeedback with other relaxation techniques, such as meditation, to enhance the self-awareness process. After biofeedback training and a period of practice, a person may be able to maintain control of the response without the machine.

Biofeedback is a common tool for treating stress-related conditions. For asthma, the particular instrument used may be an electromyograph, an instrument that measures muscle tension. When the signal indicates muscle tightening, you can use some sort of relaxation exercise, such as meditation. When the instrument indicates that the muscles have relaxed, you are on your way to learning to relax and breathing easier.

Time and cost are elements of biofeedback that a person with asthma will need to assess. Sessions last from 30 to 60 minutes once a week or daily, depending upon the individual. Recommended training takes at least 6 weeks but may stretch into weeks, months, or years. Each session can be expensive. Some insurance carriers cover biofeedback training on a limited basis.

AN ASTHMA VISUALIZATION

- Find a restful place without distraction.
- Sit in a relaxed position with your hands by your sides.
- Inhale and exhale slowly and deeply.
- Focus your mind on your breathing. Think how relaxed your breathing is and how this feeling is spreading to other muscles.
- Picture irritants or allergens that might trigger your asthma. Visualize their color and shape and how they enter your body. Follow each step of inhaling the irritant as it passes through your nose, windpipe, and lungs.
- Visualize your asthma symptoms beginning.
- Imagine that the irritants are unable to cause trouble. Suddenly, they become a less threatening shape and color.

As you counteract potential danger with positive results, you begin to relax and your breathing improves.

Movement and Breathing

YOGA BREATHING EXERCISES

Four thousand years ago in India, Hindus began practicing a physical and mental system known as yoga. A branch of yoga, called hatha yoga, developed into exercises to help believers withstand many hours of motionless meditating.

Followers in the West perform exercises to learn physical and mental control. These exercises combine deep breathing with physical poses that stretch the muscles and are usually held for about 15 to 30 seconds. Practiced with discipline over time, yoga exercises can produce considerable muscular strength and flexibility.

Studies have found some evidence that yoga is beneficial to

people with asthma. A small study of 40 adolescents showed increased lung function and capacity for exercise, fewer symptoms, and less need for medication.

You can find books to explain the basics of yoga techniques. But the best way to learn yoga positioning is through classes. Yoga classes are held in yoga centers, community recreation centers, or in YMCAs or YWCAs for a minimal cost.

T'AI CHI

T'ai chi is a Chinese system of exercise and movement (actually a martial art) designed to cultivate the flow of chi throughout the body and to give people better awareness and control over their bodies. Each exercise (there are more than 100) begins with the body in a different posture. Constant slow and deliberate movements follow, emphasizing outer movement blended with an inner stillness. T'ai chi advocates believe that by carefully exercising muscles, you create a more perfect union of body and mind.

While no studies on the effect of t'ai chi on asthma exist, studies of t'ai chi have shown that it can produce increased breathing efficiency without straining the cardiovascular system.

POSTURAL DRAINAGE

If you struggle with excessive sticky secretions that clog your airways, consider postural drainage. This is a technique performed by a therapist or trained partner to dislodge mucous plugs through gravity, forceful breathing, clapping, and vibrating. You lie in one or a series of eight different positions that correlate with the angles of the bronchial tubes. That way, each blocked lobe of the lung can drain and you can cough up excess mucus. The technique works better if performed after taking your regular medication.

With postural drainage, you first drink a large glass of water to lubricate the mucus. Then you lie on your back, stomach, or on each side. The foot of the bed is elevated about 18 inches. Your hips or other designated body parts rest on a pillow to achieve various angles. Different postures raise the affected chest area so gravity helps secretions to come forward. Sometimes, lying in one position is enough to clear your airway, if the plug site can be detected easily. Otherwise, additional positions are tried along with other techniques, such as huffing and chest clapping.

In huffing, you breathe out forcefully. At the same time, you raise and lower, or flap, one or both elbows; your arms are bent at the elbows and your hands touch your shoulders. This procedure is repeated in the drainage and upright positions.

Chest clapping can be accomplished in either position, also. This requires some help, either a therapist or someone your physician trained to know how and when to apply the technique. The partner claps various parts of your chest with a cupped hand until the mucus becomes dislodged.

Some physicians recommend using a mechanical vibrator on your chest. The vibrator quickly shakes the area in the direction of gravity, loosening the mucus. Each spot takes about a couple minutes as you exhale forcibly five times. Make sure a trained health-care professional shows your partner how to conduct the entire process and what to do should the process fail. Your condition could worsen if the procedure is performed inaccurately.

Dietary Changes

Food is essential to life. Eating a balanced diet plays an important role in general health and well-being. The right foods feed your body's organs and cells, helping them to run efficiently and grow. Poor diets that lack a balance of nutrients impair your body's ability to fight disease. Many nutrition advocates believe that diet imbalances contribute to allergen sensitivity and such chronic diseases as asthma.

Using dietary changes as a treatment option is sometimes overlooked in the medical community. Few studies, for instance, have investigated the advantages of eating one food over another to reduce asthma symptoms. Most professionals agree, however, that at least some people with allergic asthma may benefit from omitting specific foods, preservatives, and dyes from their diet that trigger allergies.

Nutrition-oriented physicians and many alternative practitioners often include dietary changes in their treatment plan. If food allergies have been identified as an asthma trigger, the only way to avoid symptoms may be to avoid certain foods. Some people may be sensitive to chemical food additives, and these are also often avoided.

Overall, dietary recommendations follow the philosophy that eating keeps the body strong enough to avert reactions to envi ronmental allergens. Although dietary changes may boost your overall health, these changes cannot cure asthma or replace medical care. Some of these recommendations make sense, particularly with specific food allergens. Others need the test of time and your patience to evaluate.

ELIMINATION DIET

Some physicians and alternative practitioners may recommend an elimination diet to discover which foods you may be sensitive to. With this diet, you eliminate a host of foods suspected as allergens. You follow a basic diet for a week or so without any additions. This gives your body a chance to eliminate any chemicals or allergy-producing agents that it has accumulated. You reintroduce one new food at a time, carefully noting in a detailed journal everything you eat, how much and when, and any aftereffects.

Once you have identified the foods you are sensitive to, a nutritionist or an allergist can help you sort out your findings and guide you in choosing what foods you add to your diet. Nutritionists can offer creative recipes for limited diets, which can keep you from losing interest in the foods while you are following the diet. Food specialists can also adapt the diet to your time constraints and budget.

Proteins are the component of food usually responsible for allergic sensitivity. Most allergens produce reactions even after they have been cooked or processed. The most common allergy-causing proteins in the US come from cow's milk, chicken eggs, peanuts, wheat, nuts, and soybeans.

How foods relate to each other and to allergies can be confusing. Nutrition experts group foods into families. Often, foods in the same family contain similar proteins. A person with allergies may find that an allergy to one food signals similar allergies—a cross-reaction—to other foods in that family. For example, if you are allergic to the cola nut, a stimulant in soft drinks, you probably cannot tolerate chocolate, either.

The concept does not always work out logically, though. If you are allergic to nuts, for instance, you may think that you need to avoid peanuts as well. But peanuts are classified in the legume, or bean, family and probably would not cause a cross-reaction.

All the foods recommended in an elimination diet will be fresh and unprocessed. Your diet might include fresh meats and fish, vegetables, grains, beans, fruits, and whole-grain breads and cereals. You could drink water, unsweetened juices, and herbal teas. As you sort out reactions to newly added foods, you learn what is safe to eat.

The elimination diet can be a long and time-consuming process. Keeping thorough enough records to follow your progress can be a chore. The elimination diet is never a replacement for medical treatment of asthma. Unless food allergy is your only asthma trigger, maintain close contact with your physician. Do not make extreme changes in your diet without consulting your doctor first. Ultimately, the best diet is one balanced with fresh, nonprocessed foods from all the food groups.

WEIGHT CONTROL

Controlled weight effects overall well-being. Maintaining a realistic weight is especially important with asthma. Children and adults find everyday activities more difficult when carrying extra pounds. People who are excessively overweight are placing an extra burden on their bodies, especially on their heart and lungs.

There is no magic program to overcome weight problems. Avoid fad diets or programs that ask you to buy expensive prepared foods. Preservatives in these foods may exacerbate asthma in sensitive individuals. Fad diets may rob your body of the balance of nutrients that maintains your health. Similarly, several diet plans sell packaged foods loaded with sugar substitutes, food coloring, and preservatives that may be asthma triggers.

HERBALISM AND BOTANICAL MEDICINE

Herbalism and botanical medicine are similar. Both involve the study and prescribing of plants for healing. Herbalists, however, define herbs as any plant with the resources to heal. They use the entire plant—roots, stems and all—to promote healing. Botanists, however, prefer to isolate the active ingredients in a plant to produce a remedy. Herbs can be derived from ferns, trees, seaweeds, or lichens. Herbalists prepare them as tablets, capsules, inhalants, lotions, ointments, suppositories, and liquids.

Plants have always been thought of as natural cures. Ancient peoples concocted remedies from plants long before there were conventional medications. Traditions from every continent included ingesting various herbs for nourishing, cleansing, and balancing the body and mind. These traditions have been handed down to the next generation and in some cases have been confirmed by scientific investigation. Many of today's medicines are derived from plants. Digitalis, for example, a

COMMONLY RECOMMENDED HERBS FOR ASTHMA AND ALLERGY

ASTHMA	ALLERGY
Ephedra: stimulates nerves, relieves inflammation of mucous membranes, opens airways	Bayberry: cleans vein congestion, reduces mucous secretions, serves as a sore-throat gargle
Lobelia: bronchodilator, clears lung congestion, helps stop smoking, reduces muscle spasm	Echinacea: stimulates immune system, lessens allergy symptoms
Mullein: reduces lung irritation	Myrrh: lessens mucous membrane irritation, stimulates immune system, kills fungi
Yerba santa: fights muscle spasms, kills fungi	Nettles: decreases mucous secretions, clears airways
	Yerba mansa: improves drainage during colds, infection, sore throat

drug used to treat congestive heart failure, is extracted from the foxglove plant. Penicillin, among the first identified antibiotics, is a product of a bread mold. Botanists have identified more than 750,000 plants worldwide. A good number of those have healing potential.

Practitioners claim that several herbs may prove helpful in relieving asthma symptoms. Their oils, nitrogen compounds, fats, proteins, and enzymes add to their medicinal value. Herbs can work in isolation or be combined for specific actions. For example, a blend of garlic, ivy, blackthorn, and blue vervain relieves spasms. See the table on page 186 for some herbs commonly recommended for asthma and allergy.

Herbalists categorize herbs according to their effect on the body. Each herb has a distinct composition. The composition of some herbs is complex, and a single herb may produce several different reactions. These are known as properties. See the table on page 189 showing some of the properties that directly apply to asthma symptoms.

Because herbs are generally not as powerful as modern medications, they tend to be slower acting. And some people find that their symptoms intensify before healing begins. This may be a serious drawback for a person with asthma.

The presence of alcohol in herbal remedies can be another roadblock. Besides water, alcohol is the second most common solution for preparing herbal extracts as liquids. Much of the grain alcohol is made from highly refined corn. Therefore, anyone who finds alcohol irritating or is allergic to corn should avoid herbal extracts made with grain alcohol. Alcohol absorbs so quickly in the system that even the smallest dose of corn provokes allergic symptoms within minutes. Since so many people in the

US are allergic to corn, there is a strong likelihood that it could aggravate your asthma.

Physicians often acknowledge the healing powers of herbs, but they note the lack of control over purity and dosages. Herbs—natural as they are—can be lethal in large doses. Herbs are often dispensed by individuals without formal medical training. Since some herbs act on body chemicals already in asthma medication, serious adverse interactions can result. *Always consult your physician before taking anything for your asthma.*

YEAST

Yeast is a type of fungus that lives harmlessly in the body. At times, yeast can cause infection in mucous membranes. Many forms of yeast are usually kept in check by bacteria that prevent their multiplying. In addition, the body fights infection through the immune system.

Often, yeasts can proliferate and produce infections, especially after taking antibiotics, corticosteroids, or drugs to suppress the immune system. A few practitioners claim that a yeast imbalance is the cause of most disease, including asthma; this condition is sometimes referred to as yeast overgrowth syndrome. They assert that positive treatment comes only after maintaining a totally yeast-free diet.

These claims are unproven to date. On rare occasions, yeast provokes lung disease. Fungus spores from outside are inhaled into the body and settle in the lungs, or organisms migrate from other organs. It is also possible to develop yeast allergies.

Physicians treat yeast infection with medications. A diet that eliminates yeast benefits people who have yeast allergy and asthma. For most asthmas, however, the yeast connection is weak.

HERBAL PROPERTIES THAT AFFECT ASTHMA

PROPERTY	ACTION	EXAMPLES OF HERBS
Analgesic	Reduces pain, congestion	Catnip, chamomile, skullcap
Antacid	Reduces excess stomach acid, calms and shields stomach lining	Slippery elm, fennel
Antiasthmatic	Helps dilate airways, breaks up mucus	Mullein, comfrey, coltsfoot
Antibiotic	Kills germs and infection, builds up immune system	Garlic, thyme, chaparral, echinacea
Anticatarrhal	Eliminates excess mucus; releases fluids through urine, sweat, feces	Cinnamon, sage, senega, anise
Antiseptic	Reduces bacteria growth	Garlic, myrrh
Antispasmodic	Relaxes muscle spasms	Rue, valerian
Astringent	Reduces swelling, decreases hemorrhaging	Calendula, myrrh, stoneroot
Demulcent	Reduces inflammation	Chickweed, marshmallow, slippery elm
Diaphoretic	Stimulates perspiration, triggers elimination, purifies body	Cayenne, ginger, peppermint
Diuretic	Stimulates urine flow, reduces swelling and inflammation	Dandelion, horsetail, nettles
Expectorant	Gets rid of excess mucus	Coltsfoot, eucalyptus, horehound, sage
Rubefacient	Reduces congestion and swelling	Cinnamon, eucalyptus, mustard seed oil
Sedative	Calms nervous system	Catnip, chamomile, passionflower, skullcap, valerian

VITAMINS AND MINERALS

Alternative treatments involving vitamins and minerals are on the rise in the US. Vitamins and minerals are essential parts of all foods, and they are critical to humans. In the body, they promote chemical reactions for releasing and using energy from food. A balanced diet usually contains enough vitamins and minerals to maintain body health. Still, even your physician may recommend vitamin or mineral supplements if your symptoms suggest a severe enough deficit to cause disease.

Researchers have isolated certain groups of vitamins and minerals that produce the greatest effects on normal body functions:

• There are 12 primary vitamins: A, C, D, E, K, and seven B vitamins, known as the B complex. These are classified into two groups: fat-soluble and water-soluble. Fat-soluble vitamins (A, D, E, and K) combine with fats from the intestine and are stored in fatty tissue for long periods.

Water-soluble vitamins (C, B_{12}, and other B-complex vitamins) remain in the body only a short time before being excreted in urine. Deficiencies of water-soluble vitamins are more likely because of their short stay. Therefore, you need to eat foods rich in water-soluble vitamins daily.

• At least 13 minerals are critical to a healthy body: chromium, copper, fluorine, iodine, iron, phosphorus, magnesium, potassium, chloride, selenium, sodium, zinc, and calcium.

• The body uses only small amounts of trace minerals, such as sulfur and manganese. Yet, scientists are researching their potential role in preventing disease.

Considerable controversy surrounds the role of vitamins and minerals as curing agents, particularly for asthma. The exact role of vitamins and minerals in preserving health is unclear, and scientists sometimes disagree about what constitutes an adequate intake. Recent studies contend that three key chemical agents are important for treating and preventing asthma: vitamin C, vitamin B_6, and magnesium.

Vitamin C. Vitamin C, or ascorbic acid, is one of the more hotly debated vitamins. In 1753, a naval physician named James Lind first noted that eating citrus fruits daily kept away the dread disease scurvy. By 1803, physicians linked vitamin C deficiency with terrible asthma attacks during scurvy. Since then, there have been a series of conflicting reports about the advantages of taking vitamin C supplements for asthma and other diseases.

Vitamin C is a water-soluble vitamin known to foster many chemical reactions in the body. It keeps teeth, bones, and tissues healthy and helps produce specific neurotransmitters, chemicals that transmit nerve cells. In addition, vitamin C acts on adrenal glands, those tiny glands above the kidney that produce natural steroids. Adrenal glands protect the body against stress, balance fluid retention, and reduce inflammation—all important activities for asthma and controlling the immune system response to infection.

Some study results showed that levels of vitamin C are lower during acute asthma episodes, establishing a loose link between them. Recent research discovered that 500 milligrams of vitamin C taken regularly resulted in increased airflow and a decrease in the number and severity of acute attacks. Researchers noticed that patients' spasms relaxed after they took vitamin C, although allergic asthma remained unaffected by vitamin C intervention.

Even with these studies, physicians caution against taking vitamin C supplements independently. Generally, a balanced diet provides all the vitamin C the body needs. Foods that are good sources of vitamin C are citrus fruits, tomatoes, green leafy vegetables, potatoes, green peppers, strawberries, cantaloupe—fresh fruits and vegetables requiring a lot of sunshine to grow. Because vitamin C is water soluble, there is little harmful buildup in the body. Still, intake of more than 1 gram can be toxic to the body. Cases of nausea, stomach cramps, diarrhea, and mental disorientation can result from self-medication with vitamin C.

Vitamin B$_6$. The chemical name for vitamin B$_6$ is pyridoxine. This vitamin commonly stimulates body chemicals that absorb carbohydrates, fats, and proteins. It is critical to the production of red blood cells and antibodies that maintain the digestive and nervous systems.

Natural healers claim that childhood asthma originates from a defect in leukotrienes, one of the many chemicals released by mast cells after exposure to an allergen. The defect causes bronchial muscles to tighten. Vitamin B$_6$ supplements are thought to block leukotriene action and reduce narrowing. After prolonged treatment, vitamin B$_6$ reduces the number and intensity of asthma attacks. This theory has not been scientifically proven.

Balanced diets usually contain enough pyridoxine. Foods that contain vitamin B$_6$ include bananas, potatoes, dried beans, wheat germ, whole grains, fish, liver, chicken, and pork. Too little pyridoxine can cause mouth and tongue swelling, skin disorders, weakness, depression, anemia, and seizures in children. Therefore, do not add pyridoxine to your diet without medical supervision.

Magnesium. Magnesium plays a vital role in several body functions. The mineral helps discharge nerve impulses, form bones and teeth, and stimulate many chemical enzymes that keep muscles, heart, and nerves working. Magnesium also directs calcium into the bones. This keeps calcium out of the bloodstream, where it could travel systemwide to cause buildup and damage.

Recent studies focus on magnesium's role in lung function. The mineral appears to block chemicals that inflame the lungs. Magnesium accomplishes this by stabilizing mast cells and T cells released during exposure to allergens. The results are relaxed airway muscles and open bronchioles that contribute to improved lung function and a reduction in wheezing and other asthma symptoms.

As with most vitamins and minerals, a balanced diet contains enough magnesium. Average daily intake of magnesium is about 380 milligrams a day. Recommended daily doses vary from 50 milligrams for newborns to 100 milligrams in young men. Women, and older people, seem to need less magnesium with age.

Foods rich in magnesium include green vegetables, whole-grain cereals and breads, soybeans, nuts, milk products, and seafood. If you are not sensitive to these foods, they may help decrease the severity of your asthma. Significant amounts of magnesium are lost in cooking and refining. Therefore, if you eat mainly processed meals, your chances of having enough magnesium in your diet are less than if you eat only whole, natural foods. Magnesium compounds are added to most antacids, so people with gastric reflux receive an added magnesium boost from their medication.

Do not prescribe magnesium supplements for yourself. Too much magnesium is just as troublesome as too little. Besides breathing difficulties, too little magnesium can cause poor calcium absorption, restlessness, tremors, and anxiety. Too much magnesium, however, contributes to nausea, vomiting, diarrhea, shakiness, and being lightheaded.

6

Asthma Emergencies

WHEN TO CALL A DOCTOR

An asthma attack is a very frightening experience. The stranglehold on your airways can make you feel as if you are drowning or suffocating. Inside, airway muscles tighten, mucous glands go into high gear, and mucous plugs gum your bronchioles.

Terrifying as an attack can be, however, appropriate treatment early in the attack will ensure that the episode runs its course without doing you serious harm. Some flare-ups, however, refuse to ease. They provoke such severe asthma that your regular treatment plan may still leave you gasping for breath. The attack may last longer than normal, or symptoms may continue to build. You need to call your physician or hospital emergency department when:

- Your peak flow drops below 50 percent of your personal best (in other words, when you are in the "red zone")
- Your short-acting bronchodilator doesn't relieve your symptoms
- Your wheezing, coughing, or breathlessness makes it difficult for you to talk
- You cannot sleep, work, or participate in recreational activities
- The skin between your ribs and your neck looks taut, indicating you are straining with your neck and rib muscles to breathe
- Your symptoms continue after you have rested
- You feel clammy and weak
- Your lips and fingernails turn gray or blue
- You are exhausted from trying to breathe

Warning: Never rely on the presence or absence of wheezing or coughing to judge the severity of an attack. Wheezes and coughs can fool you. During an attack, your airways may be so clogged that you cannot move enough air out of your lungs to produce wheezes or coughs. If your regular medication does not work, call your physician.

Prolonged attacks resistant to medications can become life-threatening. Physicians call these severe attacks status asthmaticus; they require emergency care immediately. During these severe, prolonged attacks, several dangerous body changes occur:

- Breathing speeds up (hyperventilation) to compensate for increasing lack of air

- Oxygen levels fall, weakening your system
- Carbon dioxide collects in the blood, leaving you drowsy or lightheaded
- Carbon dioxide makes your blood become acidic

If your symptoms reach this point, you may not be able to call for an ambulance yourself. If you notice these symptoms in someone else, particularly drowsiness or lightheadedness, call for emergency assistance immediately. The most common causes of death involve failure to take prescribed medications and to recognize when symptoms become seriously threatening. Most people have several hours to monitor their symptoms, test with peak flow, take medication, or call for help before they are in danger of death. About 10 percent to 25 percent of asthma deaths, however, occur in people who die within 3 hours after symptoms appear.

You and your physician need to identify what constitutes dangerous symptoms for you, what actions to take, and when to call for help. Your asthma is more threatening if:

- You required hospital or emergency department care for asthma within the last year
- Your attacks turned life-threatening, resulting in hospitalization or admission to an intensive care unit within the last year
- Your last emergency asthma attack was so severe that you needed a respirator to breathe
- You currently take, or recently stopped taking, oral corticosteroids
- You have heart disease, seizure activity, or other chronic disease in addition to asthma

- You have severe emotional problems, such as depression, alcohol abuse or problems related to alcohol abuse, or extreme anxiety
- You have allowed your disease to continue uncontrolled for 1 to 2 weeks or more. (Even individuals with moderate asthma are at grave risks if their symptoms remain unstable.)

AN EMERGENCY PLAN

Devise an emergency plan before a crisis happens. Map each asthma-related scenario that could happen with your physician. Preplanning helps avoid delays in beginning life-saving asthma treatment. Moreover, planning ahead gives you a feeling of control over your disease. Contingency plans offer you confidence that there is always something else that can be done to help you breathe easier. Here are some steps to follow in devising your emergency plan.

- **Put your emergency plan in writing.** Memory tends to falter under extreme stress, such as the stress you may experience during a severe asthma attack. You may be unable to explain to family, friends, or health-care workers what they need to know while you are in the midst of an attack. Once you finalize a plan with your physician, place the written information somewhere easily accessible to you or a family member or friend. Show your helpers where to find the written plan.
- **Add basic information to your plan, so all addresses and phone and identification numbers are handy.** Even information

you think you know well may elude you during an emergency. Include the following:

- Physician's name, telephone number, and office address
- Pharmacy name, address, and telephone number
- Hospital emergency unit name, telephone number, and address
- Insurance plan coordinator, or who to call for authorization, if you need clearance to go to a hospital emergency department, along with your insurance identification number
- Taxi service name and telephone number
- Ambulance service name and telephone number
- Relatives'/friends' names and telephone numbers

- **List medications you are taking, their timing, and doses.** Keep a list of your medications with you at all times, especially when traveling, to give to anyone providing you with medical assistance. A medication list helps emergency personnel quickly determine what else to prescribe to ease your symptoms, especially if you are unable to speak. Make sure you have a list at home and another at work.

- **Decide with your physician what steps you should take if your peak flow enters the danger zone:**

  - When to call the doctor
  - Which medication to try
  - When and how much medication to take and length of time to wait before trying another dose
  - When to go straight to the doctor's office, clinic, or hospital for emergency care

- Which relative or friend to contact for assistance and support

Determine how you will travel to the doctor or hospital. Even if you normally drive, you may not be in a position to navigate traffic safely. Decide ahead when, and under what circumstances, you should call a relative, friend, taxi, or ambulance.

- **Keep insurance or other medical information handy.** Hospitals require certain pieces of information for their own use or for insurance companies, particularly for health maintenance organizations (HMOs), other managed care plans, or for federal Medicare and Medicaid programs. Know what you need in advance. Keep your insurance card in your wallet at all times, and place an extra insurance form in your emergency packet, just in case.

Make sure your insurance company—whether HMO, preferred provider organization (PPO), or other type of organization—covers the cost of emergency department visits. Sometimes it depends upon whether the attending physician deems your visit an emergency. If the physician does not think your episode was a true emergency, you could be saddled with a hefty bill. Some managed care insurance carriers pay if your physician refers you to the emergency department and calls ahead for you. Familiarize yourself with the process for dealing with emergency care, which may differ from regular office visits and hospitalization. Know whom to call for further instructions and how to register a claim. Ask about continuing care and how referrals to specialists are made.

- **Keep your medications in their original containers and easily accessible.** You should bring every medication you take, even nonasthma medicines, to the hospital. Bringing them along leaves no doubt about your medications and their contents. Remember to include vitamins, eyedrops, nose sprays, skin creams, inhalers, and birth control and hormone patches and pills. These are medicines, too.

• **Consider obtaining and wearing a necklace or bracelet that alerts emergency personnel to your illness.** Medic Alert Foundation (see the Resources at the back of this book) offers a 24-hour worldwide emergency service in addition to inscribed jewelry. The bracelet provides the telephone number to call for additional information about you. You can give the foundation your treatment plan, list of allergies, insurance information, and any instructions about your care. When emergency treatment providers call, they receive an up-to-date report on your status. If you cannot communicate this information yourself, this report saves time and allows treatment to begin more quickly.

• **Carry a report from your last hospital or emergency visit.** Chances are high you may see a different doctor the next time around.

• **If you travel away from home, carry a doctor's summary of your treatment and medical history, insurance information, and list of medications you have taken within the past 2 weeks.** Ask if your physician can recommend a doctor or hospital at your travel destination. If you have severe asthma, carry a supply of corticosteroids in case of an acute attack. (Keep a supply at home in the medicine cabinet, too.) During an emergency, you may need a short run of corticosteroids by mouth or injection. If you have corticosteroids with you, then you can call your hometown physician to see whether the medication is necessary immediately. Precious time is not lost calling a doctor for a prescription and waiting for it to be filled.

Before leaving town, consult your physician about other details to consider on the trip, such as bringing antibiotics or nose sprays. Make sure you understand all treatment directions. Write them down to be safe.

WHAT TO EXPECT DURING EMERGENCY TREATMENT

Some people prefer to remain sick rather than seek hospital care because they fear hospitals. But asthma that does not respond to regular medication means you need professional assistance—at once. If you know what to expect, it can help reduce the stress of emergency care.

If you are experiencing an attack, try, if you can, to relax. Think about pleasant aspects of your life, such as what you will do when the attack is over to celebrate. Visualize the seashore, a walk in the forest, anything you find relaxing. Practice relaxation exercises (see pages 174 through 180) to ease your difficult breathing and the strain of what you are experiencing. Be reassured that:

- Emergency personnel know how to treat asthma and feel comfortable handling your symptoms
- Hospitals have the equipment and know-how to assess accurately the severity of your attack
- Emergency services have access to an array of medications to treat asthma quickly and effectively
- Hospitals are experienced in handling any complications that may occur (in other words, you will be in safe hands)

If possible, you, your physician, or someone helping you should call ahead to the emergency department. Hospital staff can then locate your file and be prepared with medications your physician ordered.

The goal of emergency treatment is to stabilize breathing. Therefore, expect certain swift activities to occur, beginning in the ambulance:

- You will be placed on a folding cot and wheeled into the ambulance. Your vital signs—breathing, heart rate, blood pressure—will be monitored continuously. This information will be passed along to hospital personnel.
- Your breathing will be assessed through preliminary examination.
- You will receive an inhaled bronchodilator to reduce airflow obstruction. Medication will most likely be administered by nebulizer.
- Your severe asthma may require a shot of epinephrine to quickly open airways, particularly if an allergic reaction triggered the extreme response.

At the Hospital

Once at the hospital, you will encounter many people and situations. Everything may be moving fast, since hospitals are bustling places. Each hospital emergency department follows its own procedures. Should you arrive on your own, here is some idea of what may happen.

Unless you arrive in an ambulance or are unable to speak, your first encounter will be with a receptionist who gathers information about your health and your insurance coverage. The person who accompanies you to the hospital can help you complete the forms. You may be asked to sit in a waiting area.

Be sure to let the person registering you know if you are having serious trouble breathing. Emergency personnel attend to patients according to severity of illness, rather than the order of their arrival. If you are in severe distress or arrive by ambulance, you will need treatment immediately.

Ask a nurse to contact your physician. Give your written medication list and other medical information to the doctor or nurse handling your treatment. Without written information, you will be asked many more questions before treatment can begin.

Emergency Department Care

Rooms in an emergency care unit often lack a certain degree of privacy. Many do not have four walls; instead, emergency beds are in small cubicles surrounded by curtains. Once you are situated in a cubicle, relaxation exercises may help block out sounds of other emergency room patients and staff.

A physician conducts a thorough examination in one of these cubicles. The examination focuses on assessing the severity of your illness and identifying any complications or other disease that affects your breathing, such as sinus infection, upper airway obstruction, or pneumonia. If your child has asthma, you as a parent will be able to be present during several procedures that take place during the preliminary examination:

- The physician may ask you to measure your peak flow—how fast you breathe out—and forced expiratory volume—how long and fully you exhale (see Chapter 3).
- Oxygen levels in the blood will be monitored by a pulse oximeter, a device that clips onto a fingertip or earlobe and gives a continuous reading.

- You will be given a complete blood count test if you have fever and are on corticosteroids; blood tests will check for oxygen levels, infection, and theophylline levels, if theophylline is part of your treatment. (Blood tests are one way physicians decide whether patients are so exhausted they need to be placed on a breathing machine.)

Unless you have a heart condition or other suspected lung disease, you probably will *not* receive a chest X ray.

Treatment

The frequency of breathing treatments and how often you are monitored will depend upon the severity of the attack. Hospital personnel generally follow the most recent treatment guidelines devised by the National Heart, Lung, and Blood Institute (NHBLI). These include the following:

- **Oxygen for most patients.** Usually, you will receive an oxygen mask. This will ease your breathing until medication begins to work and your oxygen blood levels increase. Levels continue to be measured by the pulse oximeter.
- **Three treatments of beta$_2$ agonists.** You can puff on your regular bronchodilator inhaler or receive medication by nebulizer with a mask. These treatments are given every 20 to 30 minutes for an hour. Thereafter, the frequency of medication varies according to improvement in your breathing. Studies indicate little difference in airflow improvement between inhaler and nebulizer delivery methods. The choice depends upon your ability to coordinate an inhaler. With either method, your heartbeat will be monitored for signs of too much bronchodilator and your medication will be adjusted as necessary.

- **Systemic (systemwide) corticosteroids.** If you have moderate or severe asthma and fail to improve enough with the initial course of bronchodilator, you will probably receive corticosteroids. This medicine will be given orally or with intravenous fluid through a needle in your arm. Either method works effectively to reduce airflow blockage and the rate of relapse.

Infants and younger children will always receive this medication to reduce the likelihood of their asthma worsening. Youngsters also tend to become dehydrated during an asthma attack. Therefore, your child with asthma will receive fluids through an intravenous tube until his or her condition stabilizes.

Throughout treatment, hospital staff will continuously monitor your progress. They will measure your blood pressure, listen to airflow in your chest, and measure your heartbeat electronically. Periodically, staff will draw blood and check the oxygen level seeping into your nose clip. Although these interruptions may be uncomfortable, this process of evaluating and reevaluating is a critical component of good treatment.

Hospital Admission

In most situations, symptoms will respond to medications within 3 hours. You may be observed a while longer to make sure your breathing remains stable. Then you will be released with corticosteroid tablets and directions about how to reduce the number you take gradually. The emergency physician will strongly recommend that you visit your own doctor for follow-up. A severe attack suggests that you need to reevaluate your original treatment plan to ensure more effective symptom control.

If your asthma fails to respond to aggressive emergency room care, you will be admitted to the hospital. Your condition is not improving if:

- Your lack of airflow indicates severe obstruction
- Your medical history reveals other severe attacks
- Your symptoms continue to deteriorate
- Your breathing is so labored you are exhausted to the point of almost losing consciousness
- You still show slight breathing difficulty and have inadequate support at home

Hospitals consider status asthmaticus a serious situation. Your physician may place you in an intensive care unit (ICU). Some ICUs are sectioned off with curtains, similar to the emergency department. Others are separate rooms monitored by machines hooked up to a central station in the hall. In the ICU, you will receive highly monitored care. Try to keep calm about needing intensive care. These precautionary measures benefit your health.

In a small percentage of admitted asthma patients, bronchial tubes almost totally close. If this happens to you, you will be placed on a breathing machine called a mechanical respirator. The doctor inserts a flexible plastic tube through the mouth and into the trachea (windpipe). The machine takes over delivering oxygen and removing carbon dioxide from the body. By breathing with a respirator, your tired lungs gain a much-needed rest and airway muscles strengthen.

As you improve, the doctor will lessen the mechanical airflow. Gradually, you will breathe on your own without the respirator. If your breathing remains stable without the respirator, you will be home within a few days. You may feel worn-out for another couple of days. Severe asthma attacks take their toll on the body.

But even people who experience repeated severe attacks can bring their asthma under control. With the right treatment plan, you can take care of almost any asthma emergency.

REASSESSING YOUR TREATMENT PLAN

While an asthma emergency is a frightening experience, it is also an opportunity to explore your past treatment—what has worked and what has not—as well as further refine your care for the future. It is important to realize that most asthma emergencies are preventable. For most people with asthma, an unexpected visit to the doctor's office or a trip to the emergency department occurs because the treatment plan developed with the doctor is not being followed or is no longer adequate.

After the emergency passes, it is important to sit down with your physician and analyze all aspects of your asthma care leading up to the emergency. Asking the following questions may be useful:

- Was this attack caused by an exposure to an asthma trigger, either one you already know about or one that is new?
- Was your asthma well controlled before the attack? Is it possible that you and your doctor underestimated the severity of your disease? In retrospect, should the dose of your inhaled corticosteroid have been larger?
- Were you taking your medications appropriately? Were you inadvertently using empty canisters?
- Was there any miscommunication between you and your doctor regarding your treatment plan or medication dose?
- Was your written action plan appropriate? Would more aggressive treatment earlier on have prevented this attack?

7

◈

Asthma and Your Lifestyle

Asthma can turn your life inside out. Planning ahead, preparing contingency programs, following medication schedules, and preventing episodes can fill your life with many details. Handling asthma extends beyond you, your treatment, and how you treat your body. Depending upon your asthma triggers, you may need to consider the weather, your environment, your job, schoolwork (if the person with asthma is your child), and other people's habits. Until you become familiar with the ramifications of chronic breathing problems, you may find dealing with asthma overwhelming. Try not to let any negative feelings about having asthma interfere with living an active, normal life.

YOUR EMOTIONS

Just the word *asthma* may evoke strong emotions in people unfamiliar with the disease. You or your child with asthma may develop strong feelings about the disease and not be entirely aware of them. Common emotional reactions to a diagnosis of asthma are fear and anxiety, frustration and anger, and depression.

Fear and Anxiety

Fear and anxiety are understandable emotions when you are faced with a chronic disease that may have unpredictable complications. You may worry that an asthma attack will surprise you in the middle of the night. You may fear that a choking episode may result in a mad dash to the emergency department. You may be concerned that the future may bring disability or even death.

Anxieties about asthma come to you or your child from several real sources, including the following:

- The physical discomfort of an attack
- Concern about experiencing symptoms or taking medication in public
- Anxiety that a severe attack may come when you are alone
- Fear that an unexpected attack may interfere with ongoing activities and performance

A healthy dose of anxiety may actually be useful. It can help you plan ahead and stay on the treatment track, avoiding asthma triggers, scheduling follow-up doctor visits, and taking prescribed medications. But too much anxiety, or too little, may have serious implications for your health.

IS YOUR ASTHMA UNDER CONTROL?

Asthma can be baffling, frustrating, and life-threatening. With so much to learn about dealing with this disease, you may find knowing where to begin difficult. Here are some questions adapted from the National Lung Association (NLA). If you can answer yes to these questions, you are on your way to controlling your asthma:

Do you have a regular physician who keeps up with the latest asthma research and treatments? ____yes ____no

Do you understand how your lungs function and how asthma is altering normal developments? ____yes ____no

Have you identified your personal asthma triggers? ____yes ____no

Do you keep a journal or have a checklist so you can learn more about your asthma patterns? ____yes ____no

Did you stop smoking or discover ways to avoid secondhand smoke? ____yes ____no

Are you aware of your early warning signs of an asthma flare-up? ____yes ____no

Have you identified what action to take once warnings begin? ____yes ____no

Did you plan in writing when and where to seek emergency medical assistance? ____yes ____no

Do you understand why you are taking each medicine and follow your doctor's prescribed treatment? ____yes ____no

Do you eat sensibly and plan a well-balanced diet that avoids foods that may cause allergies or may be asthma triggers? ____yes ____no

Is your life full and active without interferences from asthma? ____yes ____no

One or more no answers is a sign that you need to review your treatment plan and gain control of your situation.

High levels of anxiety over asthma can lead to using the condition as a crutch. You may curtail activities or remove yourself from situations you could be enjoying. You may plead helplessness and dependency out of proportion to the severity of disease. If your child has asthma, you may naturally struggle to protect him or her, then end up being overprotective. When a flare-up occurs, you may overreact, complicating your child's breathing problems with added stress.

Conversely, too little anxiety may cause you to disregard symptoms. You may mislabel or dismiss important signs of asthma, thinking they are fleeting and unimportant. You may become unrealistic about your disease. You may avoid taking preventive precautions and emergency medications or refuse to seek help, even during emergency situations.

For many people with asthma, excessive anxiety contributes to guilt feelings:

- **You worry that asthma is your fault.** Decades ago, many people believed mistakenly that individuals somehow caused their own asthma or their children's asthma. Be assured that nothing you did contributed to your asthma. You merely have supersensitive lungs. Although you have no control over your having asthma, you do possess the ability to control the disease through understanding and proper management.

- **You think that you impose on your family.** Watching someone have an asthma attack can be frightening. An interrupted family outing can be disappointing. You can lessen these disconcerting feelings among family members and allay your guilt by:

  - Helping family members understand your or your child's asthma
  - Allowing them to vent their feelings without passing judgment
  - Discussing what each person can do to help

- **You fear mounting medical bills.** Depending on your insurance coverage, your finances may become strained. Plan ahead by talking with your insurance carrier about ways to reduce your share of costs. If you have serious financial worries, consider seeing a financial planner. Investigate other insurance carriers or such government programs as Medicaid.

Frustration and Anger

Asthma can bring feelings of frustration and anger. For some, those emotions may come when their search for a "quick fix" proves fruitless. People with asthma are often surprised to learn how complicated finding the right treatment can be.

Since asthma requires care all the time, not just when symptoms flare, emotional setbacks can occur. Treatments that involve taking anti-inflammatories and bronchodilator inhalers many times a day and the additional planning to avoid triggers can be aggravating. Checking in with a physician more regularly is time consuming and expensive and can be a source of frustration.

Anger and frustration can mount as you become aware of the painful lifestyle changes that your condition will require. Perhaps asthma will affect your exercise routine, recreation choices, or job requirements. Perhaps you will need to alter everything from cleaning habits to sleeping positions—or even find a new home for the family pet.

Anger may peak with the disappointing realization that there is no complete cure. You may ask, "Why me?" or "Why my child?" You may become angry at people who are healthy and grow frustrated at what your own body is unable to accomplish. You need to help your child with asthma deal with his or her anger and other feelings about it.

Depression

Asthma can take its toll on your self-image, too. Until your symptoms are under control, you may slow down. Perhaps you have curtailed activities you once enjoyed. If you are a perfectionist, you may feel you are now less than perfect. If you normally take great pride in staying fit, you may feel upset by frequent medication doses that can be a constant reminder that you are sick. Some adults harbor fearful memories of the asthma that stalked their childhood and threatens a comeback.

These feelings can build into depression, a mental disorder that needs treatment (as opposed to the occasional bout of "the blues"). Warning signs of depression include:

- Lack of interest in normally satisfying activities
- Sleeping as an escape
- Inability to sleep
- Negative view of the world
- Desire to remain isolated from other people

Physicians are concerned that people with asthma who are also depressed may refuse to follow the prescribed treatment plan. If you are experiencing some of the warning signs of depression or a health-care provider has suggested that you may be depressed, try to be open to the possibility of getting help. Untreated depression is always a serious problem, but untreated depression in combination with asthma can be dangerous.

Taking Care of the Emotional Side of Asthma

You *can* brighten your outlook toward dealing with chronic disease. In turn, you may begin to feel better overall. If having asthma is provoking troublesome emotions, consider taking the following steps:

• **Talk with your physician.** Perhaps your medication is causing too many unpleasant side effects, altering how you cope with life and your asthma. Perhaps there are treatment options that you have not yet explored. Keeping the lines of communication open between you and your physician is the best way to ensure getting the best treatment.

• **Learn as much as you can about asthma and what your particular symptoms mean.** Knowledge can be a powerful source of reassurance that can lessen the negative impact of living with potentially serious illness.

• **Adapt the information you learn into an action plan.** Knowing what steps to take to control asthma helps reduce anxiety. Moreover, managing asthma yourself builds confidence. As you feel more confident about preventing and controlling your asthma flare-ups, your anxiety and frustration should lessen and your fears should gradually diminish.

• **Keep in mind that deaths from asthma are rare.** The few people who die from asthma usually lack proper medical care or medication. Accept that you are normal for being concerned and use this concern constructively to devise a preventive plan.

• **Allow yourself time to adjust to having a chronic disease.** You may go through feelings similar to the mourning process that people go through after losing a loved one: denial, sadness, anger. In this case, the loss may be a sense that your body is no longer invincible. Once you pass through a range of feelings, you can learn to accept your body as it is—asthma, sensitivities, and all.

• **Contact other people or groups who understand asthma and what you may be experiencing.** Having chronic illness can be isolating. Your friends and relatives may be unsure about what you can and cannot do. Rather than ask, they may leave you out of activities they view as physically demanding. Or you may be the kind of person who views asthma as punishment, preferring to bear the stigma alone, feeling no one can possibly understand.

By joining an asthma support group, you learn that you are not alone. You find people dealing with the same issues as you are, as a patient or a parent. You can share fears of another severe attack or concerns about becoming dependent on strong medication. Along the way, you learn more about your disease and how to deal with asthma. Support groups help you talk about problems with asthma, your feelings, and strategies you can use to adjust to your condition.

The Asthma and Allergy Foundation of America (AAFA), American Lung Association (ALA), and Asthma and Allergy Network (AAN; formerly Mothers of Asthmatics [MA]) offer local support groups around the country. National offices can refer you to individuals to talk with or other agencies nearby that conduct groups. Ask local hospital personnel in pulmonary rehabilitation or respiratory therapy departments if the hospital coordinates support groups.

If no group is available, you may want to arrange your own. Organize through your local AAFA or ALA chapters or contact the closest hospital about assistance in starting an asthma support or group education program.

If you cannot reverse your downward emotional spiral, you may need to seek professional help to deal with the psychological side of having asthma. You might find that strong emotions are aggravating your breathing problem or that your family circumstances are interfering with following treatment plans.

Always remember that seeking someone to assist you with personal problems is a sign of strength. It is positive indication that you know you have a problem and that you are willing and ready to take action. Equally important, your health depends upon your feeling better about yourself.

Your family may find benefits in attending therapy sessions, also. Asthma puts great strain on family time, finances, and emotions. Each person may have his or her own strong feelings in reaction to dealing with asthma. Children or spouses may resent the attention that the person with asthma receives after going through a serious attack. Asthma episodes can interfere with other family members' work and recreation. Counseling can help clear the air of everyone's negative emotions.

- **Practice relaxation exercises.** Relaxation exercises help reduce ongoing mental stress as well as the strain of asthma.
- **Discuss your asthma with others.** Family, friends, and coworkers can be wonderful sources of support once they know about your asthma, what to expect from you, and what they can do to help. Friends and family are concerned about you and your health, but they often are not sure what to do or say. Open discussion allows people to be the friends they want to be. The National Institutes of Health (NIH) suggests five factors to consider when talking with others:

1. Select an opportune time to tell someone you care about that you have asthma. For example, explain to friends and

coworkers in private at a time when you are free of symptoms.

2. Keep your discussion low-key. If you do not make a big deal out of asthma, people will not be encouraged to feel sorry for you. You do not want anyone being afraid to include you in activities, and you do not want them to treat you differently or think less of you because of asthma.

3. Explain that someone whose asthma is well controlled functions and performs just like anyone without asthma.

4. Describe what asthma is, what your symptoms include, and how you prevent them. People who understand that your coughing is not sickness will know they cannot catch asthma or any other coughing disease from you.

5. Provide details of your control plan. Explain when you might need assistance and how they could help. If you appear confident about your asthma, others will not overreact.

Always think of yourself as a regular person who happens to have asthma. Never allow someone to call you an *asthmatic,* as if asthma defines you and your capabilities. You are more than asthma. You are a vibrant, normal person who wants to lead a happy, healthy life.

THE OLDER PERSON WITH ASTHMA

With more Americans living longer and risks of asthma growing, the chances of someone over the age of 55 acquiring asthma are increasing. Each age group has its own special considerations. Older people are no different.

Be sure to have regular checkups to find any health problems before they affect, or are affected, by asthma. This is especially important if you are taking corticosteroids for asthma or any other disease. Discuss any symptoms with your physician, even those you believe unrelated to asthma. Your physician should regularly evaluate:

- Your blood for the number of blood cells, sugar levels, and potassium levels
- Your eyes for cataracts (changes in the lens of the eye that cause loss of vision) and glaucoma
- Your bones for brittleness and osteoporosis

Distinguishing Between Asthma and Other Diseases

LUNG DISEASE

By age 55, people who have smoked in the past or who still smoke may begin to show signs of lung disease. Sometimes a physician may have difficulty in discerning asthma from other respiratory conditions, such as chronic bronchitis and emphysema. With asthma, symptoms are usually reversible, unlike with other lung diseases. If you have asthma plus another lung disease, however, your breathing troubles may be more complicated.

HEART DISEASE

One of the biggest diagnostic riddles for physicians involves distinguishing heart disease from lung disease. Either condition can produce shortness of breath, chest pain, or tightening as major symptoms. With heart disease, the pain comes from the left ventricle, the main pumping chamber. When the chamber becomes blocked, blood backs into the lungs. Blockage leads to shortness of breath and possibly coughing and wheezing, much like in asthma.

Breathing difficulties can stem from heart disease and appear to be asthma symptoms. In this case, the breathing difficulties are known as cardiac asthma. If heart disease is ruled out, however, most physicians check further for lung disease.

Other Age-Related Conditions

Describe any other physical problems to your physician that could interfere with your ability to take medicine. These problems may be important factors if you need emergency treatment. Make sure you, a family member, or your physician alert other health-care providers to these conditions. Following are some examples.

HEARING LOSS

If you cannot hear enough to understand directions, you need to let people know. Ask your health-care provider to talk louder. If your hearing loss is severe, request that your instructions come in writing. Keep a note with you at all times that says you cannot hear. In an emergency, health-care workers may not have the time to consider whether hearing or other factors are contributing to your unresponsiveness. They may assume your condition is worse than it is because you are unable to respond, or they may view you as incapable of thinking clearly enough to handle decisions about your care. Similarly, if you are admitted into the hospital, ask for a coded sign attached to your bed that alerts staff to hearing impairment.

ARTHRITIS

Some people with arthritis find their inhaler easier to use with a spacer. Should your arthritis make coordinating a metered-dose inhaler (MDI) impossible, request medicine through a nebulizer or in a longer-acting pill form.

VISION PROBLEMS

Your physician can recommend several options to help you carry out treatment with reduced vision:

- Color-code your peak flow meter to match the levels of severity outlined in Chapter 3 (see pages 78 through 83). Differentiating tiny numbers can be difficult for someone with poor eyesight.
- Ask for instructions and information in larger type.
- Bring a tape recorder to your office visit to record treatment directions. (Tape recordings are also helpful if you have memory problems.)
- Always wear your glasses when measuring peak flow and medication doses. Keep a magnifying glass handy to read medicine bottle labels.
- Ask for a coded note attached to your hospital bed indicating vision loss, in case you are admitted following an emergency.

MEMORY

An inconsistent memory affects everyone at some time. For older adults, however, memory loss is more common. With periodic memory lapses, many older adults find it more difficult to remember medication schedules.

If memory is your problem, your physician may suggest one or more of the following actions:

• **Taking longer-acting medication.** Taking longer-acting medications means you have to take them once or twice a day, instead of four or more times. Take medication at the same specific times each day, such as before brushing your teeth or going to bed at night, to help aid your memory.

• **Buying devices to help your memory.** Pillboxes labeled with days or months, or a prepared calendar with complete treatment instructions, may help.

• **Keeping detailed written instructions.** Post instructions in an obvious spot near your medication.

• **Using a daily check-off sheet for you to note each time you take your medicine.** That way, you do not need to remember how many doses you already took.

SURGERY AND ASTHMA

At some time, you may require surgery for a health condition other than asthma. For the person with asthma, the threat of complications involving the lungs significantly increases. Nevertheless, you do have options that can ensure that your surgery runs smoothly.

Nonemergency Surgery

BEFORE SURGERY
Communicate with your regular physician, surgeon, and anesthesiologist, the doctor responsible for administering your drugs

during surgery, ahead of the surgery date. Everyone must be aware that you have asthma. The anesthesiologist in particular needs to know exactly which medicines you take and whether your asthma is under control.

If the surgery is not an emergency, your physicians will have time to review your medical history and conduct pulmonary function tests to assess your breathing. From these assessments, your physicians will determine what steps need to be taken around and during the time of your surgery. Special care is needed if:

- Your asthma treatment involves oral corticosteroids
- You recently received asthma emergency treatment
- You already experienced asthma complications with prior surgery
- You have allergies to medications
- Your surgery involves the chest or upper abdomen
- Your asthma is complicated by heart disease

People with asthma can safely undergo surgery with proper care and appropriate treatment. If your lung function is not at its best, however, your physician may recommend postponing surgery until it improves. During surgery with general anesthetic, a tube is inserted into the windpipe. The tube connects to a respirator that allows you to breathe mechanically. Sometimes, inserting the tube triggers throat reflexes that lead to bronchospasm in someone with asthma. Therefore, taking the time *before* surgery to make sure your asthma is well controlled is essential.

DURING SURGERY

You may be asked to inhale your bronchodilator just before surgery to avoid constriction during the operation. The anesthesiologist may also give you inhaled bronchodilators during the procedure. If you are on long-acting medications, you may receive them intravenously to maintain relaxed breathing.

If your lung function still remains unstable, your physician may suggest a local rather than general anesthetic. With a local anesthetic, just the surgical site on your body is anesthetized to deaden feeling where surgery takes place. You remain awake throughout the operation, although you receive medications to relax you. The wrong medication could trigger airway sensitivity, so make sure you indicate *any* medication sensitivity to the anesthesiologist beforehand.

AFTER SURGERY

You will probably be monitored more closely after surgery than someone without asthma. Fortunately, complication rates from surgery are low. Your normal asthma treatment schedule will resume as soon as your breathing stabilizes after surgery. Planning between you and your physicians can ensure a good recovery.

Emergency Surgery

If you require emergency surgery, steps you take ahead of time can help you. Risk of emergency surgery is another good reason to:

- Wear a medical alert bracelet with information about your asthma and medications
- Have your asthma medical history on file at the hospital emergency care unit
- Keep your insurance information and physician's telephone number with you at all times

PREGNANCY AND ASTHMA

Pregnancy is a time of great joy. If you are pregnant and have asthma, however, you may naturally worry about asthma's affecting your baby's chances of a safe development and delivery. You grapple with whether your body can handle the added load of pregnancy along with asthma.

Be reassured that statistics are in your favor. Asthma is one of the most common problems during pregnancy, so you are not alone. The condition affects about 1 in every 100 pregnant women. Yet, serious complications account for only 4 percent to 6 percent of all asthma pregnancies. Similar to surgery and other health considerations, however, pregnancy with asthma requires extra planning and care.

Controlling Your Asthma

Asthma that is under control rarely affects your health or the health of your baby. You breathe easily, taking in enough oxygen to energize a body of increasing size. In turn, you nourish the growing fetus by pumping oxygenated blood into the placenta, the fluid-filled sac holding the baby.

When your asthma is not controlled, oxygen levels can diminish, decreasing the fetus's life-sustaining nourishment and threatening normal development. Pregnant women with unstable asthma are more likely to experience high blood pressure, vaginal bleeding, tissue swelling, and complicated labor. Their babies are at greater risk for premature birth and lower birth weight. Both can damage a baby's health. Therefore, your physician will encourage you to continue treatment that you followed before you became pregnant—for your well-being and the baby's.

Pregnancy affects each woman differently. About one third of women report their asthma worsens. Another third find improvement during pregnancy, while the last third have symptoms that remain unchanged. For some women, pregnancy is their first exposure to asthma. Increased progesterone levels quicken respiration, causing shortness of breath.

Those who experience breathing difficulties report a rise in severity between 29 and 36 weeks (seventh and ninth months) of pregnancy. This is partly due to pressure against the lungs as the baby grows larger. Women normally encounter breathlessness during the last trimester of pregnancy. You can imagine the added burden of narrow, mucus-filled airways.

For unexplained reasons, many women find their asthma improves during labor and delivery. Should a severe attack occur during labor, your physician can help your breathing without hurting your child. About 3 months after the baby is born, pregnancy breathing patterns usually return to their prepregnancy state.

Be sure your physician or midwife knows you have asthma. If this person is different from your asthma doctor, coordinate treatment between the two. Discuss which medicines you take for asthma and whether they could harm a baby's development. If your asthma is stable, you may be able to lower doses or switch to different medication.

Make sure you follow your regular treatment plan:

- **Monitor your breathing with a peak flow meter.** Contact your physician if you notice any changes. If you are concerned about enough oxygen reaching the fetus, your physician can test oxygen levels in the blood with a blood test or by pulse oximetry, the clip that attaches your fingertip to a measurement device.

- **Avoid your asthma triggers.** You may find either that you are more sensitive to known triggers or that other substances bother your asthma during various stages of pregnancy.
- **Stay physically fit.** Eat a balanced diet and continue a moderate exercise plan. Save major changes in your exercise routine or diet until *after* the baby is born. (These guidelines are beneficial for any pregnant woman.)
- **Avoid severe winter illness by receiving a flu shot.** Get a shot with a dead (rather than live) vaccine early in the season. Flu vaccination helps prevent serious infection in the presence of moderate to severe asthma.
- **Maintain your medication schedule.**

Medications

Asthma medications can be a concern during pregnancy. You may need higher doses to maintain healthy breathing as your weight increases with the baby. Any medication you take during pregnancy crosses the placenta and affects the fetus.

The greatest concern of birth defects comes during the first 3 months of pregnancy when the baby's organs form. Thereafter, medication can slow the baby's growth rate. Delayed growth contributes to low birth weight and a host of other problems.

Unfortunately, not enough research has been done to determine the absolute safety of medications during pregnancy. Current studies show few proven adverse effects from asthma medications (see table on page 228). Carefully weigh the risks from medications with the greater threat of reduced oxygen to you and the developing baby.

Long-term treatment should probably continue during pregnancy. Some medications require modification to reduce negative effects on the baby. For example, intravenous theophylline offers benefits during an emergency. Yet, the drug can speed a fetus's heart rate and prolong delivery if dosage is too high. Your blood levels should be monitored regularly for theophylline.

Proving which medications are safe during pregnancy and which are not may take years. In the meantime, these are the allergy/asthma medications that the National Heart, Lung, and Blood Institute (NHLBI) recommends you avoid during pregnancy:

- **Live virus vaccines.** Killed virus vaccines are acceptable.
- **Immunotherapy.** Continue with allergy shots only if they help reduce your asthma. Discontinue therapy at the first sign of generalized adverse reactions. These could induce unexpected labor. Do not begin, or increase, doses of allergy shots during pregnancy.
- **Antihistamines and decongestants.** These medicines decrease excess mucus during colds and allergies. However, several cold remedies decrease blood flow to the baby during pregnancy. Decongestants made with pseudoephedrine can cause abnormal fetuses. Adrenaline compounds such as epinephrine, isoproterenol, phenylpropanolamine, and phenylephrine can cause abnormal embryo development in animals.

Some of these ingredients are in diet pills and nose sprays. Many people forget that these substances are in medications, too,

ASTHMA MEDICATIONS AND PREGNANCY

MEDICATION	USE	RISKS
Theophylline	Emergency benefits; safe at low doses; requires blood level checks	Infants born with jitteriness, vomiting, and rapid heartbeat from mother with high theophylline levels; prolonged labor and increased blood loss; increased abnormalities; greater risk of infant jaundice
Cromolyn sodium	Preferred anti-inflammatory during pregnancy	Considered safe
Bronchodilators	Used in inhalant, nebulizer, and oral forms; oral terbutaline used to prevent labor in third trimester	Considered safe
Corticosteroids	Treat severe attacks	Inconclusive results from studies on humans to date; low birth weight; premature births when taken over the long term; deformed bones with oral forms; not first-line choice during pregnancy

and they should not be taken during pregnancy. Contact your physician before taking anything that could harm your baby.

• **Antibiotics.** Several antibiotics clearly harm the fetus. Tetracycline damages fetal tissue affecting bones and teeth. Sulfa drugs are poisonous to newborns, and reports warn against ciprofloxacin and aminoglycosides, also. Ask your physician for names of products made from these chemicals, and avoid them.

• **Expectorants and cough medicines.** Iodides in liquid and tablet expectorants may alter breathing of newborns.

BREAST-FEEDING AND ASTHMA

Breast-feeding presents more choices to weigh for the woman with asthma. On one side are the benefits of nursing—reduced chances of allergies, added immunity from disease, and bonding between mother and child. On the other side are the risks of asthma medications' seeping into breast milk.

Studies report most asthma medications are safe during breast-feeding. Inhaled medicines sprayed directly into the lungs are safest because so little medicine circulates through the body to wind up in breast milk. Doctors believe that other medications enter breast milk in such small doses that only a minute amount reaches the baby. The few confirmed cautions involve taking iodides, tetracycline, and corticosteroids while breast-feeding. Reports indicate that theophylline may cause irritability in babies, but more studies are needed for verification.

If you notice unusual fussiness, stomach upset, or prolonged crying in your breast-fed baby, contact the physician. Your medication may be affecting your baby. Discuss eliminating a medication to test whether it eases the baby's discomfort. With well-controlled asthma, you may be able to adjust your medication. Or you may want to consider feeding your infant from a bottle, just to be safe.

EXERCISE AND ASTHMA

A generation ago, people who had asthma were cautioned against participating in exercise and athletic competition. Consequently, most asthma sufferers remained inactive, and their health deteriorated as a result. Poor physical health translated into lungs that were less prepared to respond to everyday strains of life.

Today, health-care professionals understand the benefits of exercise for the mind, heart, and all the body's systems. Physicians encourage everyone, including individuals with asthma, to participate in some regular physical exercise.

Almost 8 million Americans experience asthma symptoms from exercise. But that does not stop young and old athletes with asthma from exercising. Many of these people take exercise very seriously. About 10 percent of Olympic athletes exercise strenuously in spite of breathing difficulties. Perhaps you know some of these athletes with asthma:

- **Nancy Hogshead.** A three-time Olympic gold-medal swimmer who stopped competing in 1984, Nancy Hogshead believed in exercise for people with asthma enough to write the book *Asthma and Exercise* and create an exercise videotape.
- **Jackie Joyner-Kersee.** A basketball all-American and college track star, Jackie Joyner-Kersee went on to win silver and gold Olympic medals for heptathlon multievents in 1988 and 1992, when she broke her own long-jump record set at the earlier event.
- **Tom Dolan.** Tom Dolan set three US National Collegiate Athletic Association (NCAA) swimming records and was the youngest male member of the US team to swim at the Olympics in 1995.

- **Dominique Wilkins.** Dominique Wilkins's basketball playing landed him on the Atlanta Hawks and the 1987, 1988, 1990, and 1991 National Basketball Association (NBA) all-star teams.

- **Barbara Johnson.** In 1996, Barbara Johnson, mother to actor-producer Christopher Reeve, was a 64-year-old rowing champion at Boston's nationally known 1-day regatta named Head of the Charles.

- **Virginia Gilder.** Virginia Gilder was a member of the 1984 US women's rowing team that earned a silver medal. The year Gilder competed in the Olympics, 41 of the 75 US medal winners reported exercise-induced asthma. Other athletes in that competition who had exercise-induced asthma included Alexi Grewal (won a gold medal for men's road cycling), Jeanette Bolden (earned a gold medal for women's 4 × 100-meter relay), and Sam Perkins (played basketball on the US gold-medal team and went on to play professional basketball with the Dallas Mavericks.

Even though exercise can trigger asthma, physicians find that enhanced physical fitness actually helps control respiratory disease. A fit body breathes easier under stress. Less stressful breathing reduces the usual airway cooling and drying that characterizes workouts.

Studies of treadmill runners have revealed that asthma attacks begin about 6 to 8 minutes into exercise and peak about 5 to 6 minutes after exercise. Runners in the study who stopped before 6 minutes often averted symptoms. Those able to continue found their symptoms eventually eased. Similar experiments led researchers to conclude that repeated but interrupted exercise improves asthma.

The more you exercise, the greater the level of exercise required to provoke an attack. With time and gradual buildup, exertion actually decreases the risk of attack. You just need to exercise safely to gain the benefits of better breathing without the drawbacks of exercise-induced asthma.

Exercise Medications

Usually, when asthma requires a bronchodilator inhaled daily, physicians bump up patients to the next intensive treatment step for preventive medicine before exercise. Athletes with exercise-induced asthma may benefit from two extra bronchodilator puffs 15 minutes before each practice. Since exertion can cause asthma symptoms, treatment focuses on the specific trigger—exercise.

Discuss this option with your physician. Some doctors prefer to increase doses of tablets instead for someone who exercises heavily. Medication decisions with exercise-induced asthma depend upon your overall fitness, the environment where you exercise, and the frequency and extent of exercise.

Be alert to the reason for symptoms during exercise so that you do not miss signs of worsening asthma. Ask yourself whether you would need this extra medication boost if exercise were not a factor. If your response is no, then you can probably continue with your regular treatment plan, including extra puffs before exercise, without worrying about more severe asthma. If the answer is yes, your asthma may be unstable, and you need to contact your physician.

MEDICATIONS TO CLEAR NASAL PASSAGES
Air into your lungs is filtered, warmed, and humidified in the nasal passages. If you exercise with blocked upper airways, this

filtering system breaks down. Greater amounts of cooler air with pollutants, irritants, and allergens pour into the lungs. With each quickened breath, your exposure to substances that trigger chest tightness, coughing or wheezing, and breathlessness increases.

Physicians disagree about whether people with asthma should take medications to control nasal stuffiness. Some recommend taking medications before exercise to clear nasal passages and sinuses. Others claim decongestants are unnecessary, even damaging. They assure athletes that a stuffed nose should not be a problem: most people breathe through their mouth during exercise anyway.

Those same physicians are equally negative about antihistamines that dry mucus. They fear that drying thickens mucus, which blocks airways and interferes with airflow even more. Before exercising, ask your physician about antihistamines, decongestants, nasal cromolyn sodium, or corticosteroid nose sprays in addition to your regular asthma medications.

PRECAUTIONARY MEDICATION

If you exercise outdoors and react fiercely to specific pollens or stinging insects, carry injectable epinephrine. Injections are imperative for severe emergency attacks when you need fast-acting medication. Always try to exercise with someone else. Another person should be available to inject you with medication in an emergency or call for emergency assistance if you are unable to help yourself.

BANNED MEDICATION

In an effort to keep athletes from medicating themselves to enhance performance, NCAA and Olympic rules include a list of banned substances. Many medicines that help breathing are on the lists. Several top athletes have had difficulty both in qualifying for events and in breathing without medication that works best for them.

In 1972, swimmer Rick DeMont earned an Olympic gold medal for the 400-meter freestyle. But he lost his medal after officials realized that his asthma medication was a banned substance. The rules about allowable medications have been revised and most asthma medications are now permitted. The 1996 Olympic committee allowed two swimmers with asthma, Jessica Foschi from the US and Samantha Riley of Australia, to compete in spite of failing drug tests.

If you compete athletically, you should check competition rules about medication before you play. Discuss concerns with your physician. Perhaps a doctor's note and a second-opinion physical examination will be enough to satisfy the rules and maintain your quality of breathing.

Exercise Choices

You can safely participate in any form of exercise as long as your asthma is under control. Certain sports, however, arouse fewer symptoms of exercise-induced asthma. Sports that involve short spurts of exercise allow lungs to rest between exertions. They cause fewer muscle spasms than exercise that forces you to move continuously, such as long-distance running. Less demanding exercise minimizes strain on the lungs, prompting fewer asthma symptoms. (See table on page 236.)

Indoor water sports offer the greatest exercise benefits. Not only do water sports involve the entire body, but the warm, humid environment limits the airway drying and cooling that normally occurs during exercise. Most underwater sports are safe for swimmers with asthma, also. Swimming, snorkeling, and diving outdoors in warm water provide equally safe fun.

Talk with your physician before scuba diving, however. Scuba diving with breathing difficulties can cause a pressure injury known as barotrauma, which can be fatal. When a diver plunges under water, outside pressure builds as the volume of air inside the lungs drops. The danger comes when you rise after inhaling from the scuba tank. Water pressure decreases suddenly as the air inside your lungs expands. In lungs narrowed from asthma, the increased volume of air becomes trapped. Eventually, lung tissue may burst, releasing air bubbles into the bloodstream. Air bubbles that travel to the heart or brain can prove deadly.

Where to Exercise

The safest place to exercise is indoors where the air is warm and humid, such as at an indoor swimming pool. Indoor exercise keeps ozone, pollen, and sulfur dioxide pollution outdoors, so breathing comes easier.

If you must exercise outdoors, follow these guidelines:

• **Stay away from high-traffic areas.** Quiet residential streets or country roads have fewer cars and factories emitting polluted gases into the air.

• **Schedule activity during non–rush hour times, when pollution is lower.** Cancel exercise plans if there is a smog alert.

• **Perform your activity late in the day if pollens affect your breathing.** Early morning awakens flowers and grasses,

EXERCISE CHOICES AND ASTHMA

LESS STRESSFUL EXERCISE	MORE STRESSFUL EXERCISE
Swimming	Running
Walking	Ice skating (cold)
Fishing	Aerobic dancing
Golf	Basketball
Slow bicycling	Soccer
Baseball	Snow skiing (cold)
Horseback riding (unless you are allergic to horses)	Tennis

sending greater quantities of pollen into the air. Stay indoors if pollen counts are high.

- **Plan to use exercise paths away from fields full of grasses and weeds.**
- **Change your exercise path if necessary.** Avoid flower beds, flowering fields, or garbage where stinging bugs may lurk.
- **Avoid areas where water collects and molds may grow.**

Exercise Precaution Checklist

Here are precautions you should take before exercising:

- Check with your physician before starting any new or accelerated exercise program. If shortness of breath limits your exercise tolerance, begin slowly, with such exercise as walking. Walking strengthens muscles while increasing endurance for other sports. It is an exercise that travels easily and that can be increased with your stamina.

- Do not exercise when you feel sick or exhausted.

- Warm up for 15 minutes with continuous moderate exercise before and after strenuous activity, such as aerobics or jogging. Studies indicate that slow warm-up gradually saps the chemicals that signal bronchial muscles to constrict. By the time heavier activity begins, your body is prepared to exercise. Warm-ups and cool downs alleviate drastic temperature changes in the lungs that can trigger bronchial muscle tightening.

- Allow 15 to 30 minutes for bronchodilators to activate in your body before beginning exercise.

- Tell your team coach about your physician's orders so that everyone understands your condition. Let teammates know that you take medications to control asthma. Teammates can be a source of support, and they can assist you in an emergency.

- Avoid wearing perfumes, scented lotions, or brightly colored clothing that may attract stinging insects. Bees, wasps, and yellow jackets in particular can pose serious threats to allergic airways that swell immediately upon your body's receiving stings from these insects.

- Drink small amounts of fluids during exercise. You want your airways to stay hydrated to guard against mucous plugs and muscle tightening.

- Try to breathe slowly through your nose while exercising to warm air before it enters the lungs. Remember to cover your nose and mouth with a scarf or filter mask during cold weather or in high-irritant areas.

- Measure airflow with your peak flow meter if you have any doubts about the effects of exercise on your asthma. Do not be surprised to see a drop of 15 percent or more following exercise. Symptoms should respond to the discontinuation of exercise or the inhalation of medication. Should your peak flow hover at a lower point or you notice any other changes, contact your physician.

- Use your bronchodilator at the first sign of asthma symptoms.
- Exercise daily to maintain strength and increase endurance.

YOUR CHILD WITH ASTHMA

When a child has asthma, everyone in the family shares the stresses, schedules, and emotions of living with chronic disease. Controlling your child's asthma relies on the support of parents, siblings, childcare providers and sitters, school personnel, coaches, and anyone else in contact with your child regularly. You, as primary caregiver, and your physician devise and regularly update plans that help everyone involved understand what having asthma means for your growing child.

Making adjustments for individual differences is part of family life. Asthma is a minor but critical characteristic that must be accommodated in a family member. With asthma, however, you need more advance planning, emergency alternatives, and added time for preventive cleaning, doctor's visits, and other arrangements.

Infants With Asthma

It is unusual for a child younger than 2 years to have asthma or allergy problems. Caring for infants who do have asthma is challenging. Since infants' lungs function differently than older children's, it is more difficult to give them inhaled medications. Infants do let you know when something bothers them, but they cannot help you discern breathing problems from other discomfort until they are older. Thus, you must be extra alert when breathing difficulties are suspected. Share any concerns with your physician. More investigative testing may allay your fears. If asthma is confirmed, knowing how to handle your baby in an emergency will be reassuring.

To test for asthma, your baby's doctor will follow similar procedures as those used with older children and adults. You will be asked about the baby's family and medical histories, and the baby will receive a complete examination, possibly with diagnostic blood, mucus, and X-ray tests, for signs of illness. About 80 percent of early asthma comes from allergy causes.

Should your infant have asthma, try not to allow the diagnosis to cloud the relationship between you and your child. Disease adds to the normal insecurity and anxiety of caring for someone so young. As your confidence with handling an infant grows, so will your ability to manage asthma. Remember: you did not cause your baby's asthma. Moreover, understand that your baby is more than his or her diagnosis and needs the same amount of love, play, and stimulation as any child.

To reduce your anxiety, keep regular appointments with your child's physician. Work out a specific treatment plan together for handling symptoms. Learn the warning signs of infant asthma and what you can do to prevent and help your child. Devise an emergency control plan that includes traveling to the hospital or doctor, health-care payments, and supervision for your other children on a moment's notice. Make sure your child's sitters know where to find this information and medication. They need to understand the plan and when to contact you, the doctor, or emergency assistance.

The NHLBI offers these suggestions for when to seek emergency care for your infant:

- The baby's breathing rate increases to over 40 breaths per minute while the baby is asleep. To calculate your baby's rate, count the number of breaths in 15 seconds. Multiply by 4. Remember that babies normally breathe faster than older people, so try not to camp at your baby's bed counting continuously. Once you become adjusted to a baby's normal breathing, you will learn to relax.
- Your baby suddenly stops suckling or feeding.
- The infant's skin pulls tightly between the ribs with breathing, which may indicate straining to breathe.
- The baby's chest expands, swelling with air that cannot be exhaled.
- The baby's face pales or turns red or fingernails turn blue for an extended time.
- Your baby's cry changes in quality, either softening or coming in shorter gasps or as grunting sounds.
- The baby's nostrils widen and flare.

The most important thing to remember with infants who have breathing problems is to stay calm and find emergency care quickly. If you suspect your baby is experiencing severe breathing difficulties, do not:

- Offer your infant large volumes of liquid to drink, thinking the problem will wash away

- Hold a bag over your baby's nose or mouth in an effort to trap cleaner air for your baby to breathe
- Give your infant any medication—cold remedy or antihistamine—without checking with your physician first

Your Growing Child With Asthma

Like any child, your boy or girl with asthma has strengths and weaknesses and a jumble of feelings. Asthma frequently confuses these normal elements of development. Some parents compound the problem by becoming overprotective, denying that the asthma exists, or holding the child with asthma to different standards for fear punishment or excitement will trigger an episode.

This behavior skews children's concepts of themselves and their disease. Young children understand they cannot have the fun, food, or activities they may want. They may dislike doctor visits anyway. With asthma, they have even more appointments, possibly due to the need for monitoring medicine or receiving painful allergy shots or to catching more infections. Youngsters show their displeasure with tantrums, hyperactivity, lethargy, or irritability. Sometimes, these symptoms are difficult to separate from a child's normal responses to situations or reactions to medication.

As children mature, they can tell you more. But there still may be hidden feelings of frustration and anger. Children with asthma may feel they are denied fun activities and favorite foods. They encounter imposing schedules and frustrating restrictions. They become discouraged by their lack of energy, and they become frustrated by medication regimens.

Older children crave less dependency, not more because of illness. Pent-up feelings build into anger at themselves for not being healthy, anger at doctors for not fixing the asthma, and anger at family members who keep them from things they like.

Your child may also worry and have fears. Perhaps your child has already experienced the scare of severe asthma attacks. In the rush of emergency care, your child might not understand that these preventions and interventions will reverse asthma's stranglehold on his or her airways. Seeing the concern of everyone else, your child fears the disease may be worse than it is. If your young child views life in black or white, the child may even conclude that he or she will not have a long life. Reassure your child that adhering to a treatment plan will help him or her live a healthy life.

Your Teen With Asthma

Ingrained fear of attacks may immobilize the teen with asthma. Rather than risk another episode, the teenager holds back from all activity, exercise, and social events requiring exertion. Some children feel guilty that their disease interferes with so many family activities. They see mounting medical bills, interrupted vacations, and siblings vying for attention. They may feel ashamed of causing added stress with emergency visits to the hospital. Parental expectations that are different from those for siblings isolate children with asthma even more. Or they assume their asthma is punishment for bad behavior.

Your child may also feel embarrassment. Nothing bothers a preteen or teenager more than being different. An asthma episode can make a teen feel as if she or he stands out. People stare without knowing what is happening or what they can do to help. The young teen with asthma may be unable to express what is happening.

Older children may have a greater understanding of their asthma. But they may actively ignore symptoms, hoping not to make a scene. Their form of rebellion may be to test the limits of their body and their disease—an illness that can infringe upon their emerging independence and adulthood.

Another source of teenage embarrassment comes from long-term corticosteroid therapy. Corticosteroid-dependent teens must sometimes contend with bloated faces and bodies. Painful joints and brittle bones make athletics and exercise difficult. Missing school days for sickness can interfere with completing schoolwork and maintaining good grades.

Siblings and Asthma

Creating sibling harmony is a challenge for any parent. Siblings of all ages naturally compete for attention and individual recognition. When a brother or sister has chronic disease, however, the normal rules of one-upmanship change. Even the most understanding sibling may eventually resent the concern, time, and treatment involvement heaped upon a sibling who has asthma.

Reactions differ with sibling ages and the severity of asthma. Jealousy from feeling left out is a common reaction at any age. Children may resent spontaneously being shunted off to a neighbor or sitter during an emergency attack. They may dislike staying home because their brother or sister is too sick for a family outing.

Younger children may become mischievous or act out to gain their own attention. By school age, siblings may openly resent feeling neglected. They may pick fights at home or at school, thinking any attention is better than none.

Secret fears may creep in at any age. Many arise from misunderstanding. Some children fear their parents love the sick child more because that is who receives the extra attention. Healthy siblings fear they will cause an asthma episode by being nasty to or angry at their sick sibling. They see a brother or sister gasping for air and worry that he or she may die. Or they worry about catching asthma themselves. Some siblings feel guilty for being healthy.

Parents of a child with asthma can improve life with the chronic disease and educate the entire family about asthma. Understanding gives everyone the tools to work together better. Parents, children, and siblings need clear information about asthma and how they can help prevent episodes at home. When everyone participates in treatment, individuals realize their special role in the family. Here are some suggestions:

- Learn your child's triggers and remove them from the home.
- Monitor your child's behavior following the introduction of new medication. Write down the effects, positive or negative, to report them to your physician. Watch for changes in behavior, activity level, sleeping and eating patterns, coordination, and sensitivities, in addition to the extent of control over asthma symptoms.
- Understand that asthma may complicate the delicate sibling balance. Help your child with asthma understand that nothing he or she did caused the disease. Reassure your healthy child that asthma is not contagious. As a parent, you may need to work

harder to help your children recognize they, too—not just the sibling with asthma—are special. Schedule a special activity or discussion time with each child. Assign household responsibilities to each child, including the son or daughter with asthma. Communicate with your healthy children after each asthma episode to reassure them of your love.

• Teach your child with asthma age-appropriate self-care. For example, preschoolers can monitor breathing with color-coded peak flow meters. Link medication schedules to regular daily events, such as breakfast and bedtime, so your child takes at least some responsibility for remembering and taking them.

• Talk about what happened before, during, and after each asthma episode, so your child learns to associate triggers with episodes and learns about interventions that prevent worsening asthma. Stress the fact that asthma symptoms cannot be ignored. Tell your child to stay calm and seek adult assistance whenever asthma symptoms begin. If no adult is nearby, teach your child to call 911 or other emergency numbers in your area. Have your child write an asthma plan, including triggers and medications. Cut out pictures or use stick figures to visualize options, if your child cannot write. Teach your child relaxation exercises, too (see pages 174 through 180).

• Gradually, encourage your child to establish a relationship with the physician, monitor his or her own health, and schedule follow-up care independently. The more your child understands what is happening to his or her body, the better the child can contend with difficulties. With your guidance, your maturing child learns that any feelings will be heard. Increasing personal responsibility helps improve overall problem solving, confidence, and a more positive self-image.

- Encourage participation in physical activities, exercise, and sports.
- Role-play different aspects of asthma. Have your child with asthma act out an attack and the actions to be taken in response. Younger children can practice calling for help, doing relaxation exercises, and administering medication to a doll or stuffed toy. Watch that your child uses a peak flow meter and inhaler correctly. Help your child practice speaking up and refusing politely when unknowing adults offer tasty treats that trigger allergies.
- Share with your child books and videotapes about children who have asthma and how they learn to feel better. Stories help children understand that others have similar reactions and concerns. Some recommendations are listed in the Resources section at the back of this book.
- Role-play between siblings. Acting gives children the opportunity to express their feelings in a nonjudgmental environment and discover alternatives to deal with emotions.
- Give siblings a realistic view of asthma. Siblings can learn what they can do to help at home. Let them know that everyone is special, whether he or she is sick or not. The child with asthma may have specific health concerns to deal with, but reassure healthy siblings you are always available for them, too.
- Remember that your teenager's hiding symptoms from the public—or you—is different from denying the disease. One study found that teens who worry less and conceal their asthma symptoms perceive their disease more accurately and control symptoms better.
- Consider offering your child with severe asthma the chance to go to an asthma camp. While there is nothing about asthma that demands isolating your child, a camp with other children

who have asthma may produce lasting benefits. Fun activities are geared to individual energy levels. Trained staff help children learn to take better care of their breathing. Children meet other children like themselves. They learn they are not alone, and they find out they are not so different after all. Such realizations can build confidence.

• Seek professional intervention if unresolved family stresses become so serious they interfere with asthma treatment. Community organizations may offer individual or group family counseling on a sliding fee basis, which can be affordable. Asthma and stress go together poorly: one augments the other. Better to reduce family tensions, so that the whole family can deal with asthma.

• Be a health-care role model for your children. Study results show that children mimic their parents' attitudes toward illness, even if parents are not asthmatic. If you deal with disease symptoms realistically—a balance between not being self-conscious yet not being in denial—your children will judge asthma symptoms more accurately.

Asthma at School

Asthma is the leading cause of school absences. Missing school might sound great to some students. But to children with asthma, attending school signifies good health and stable asthma. To achieve both, once again you need to plan ahead—this time with your child's school.

Education is a two-way street with school personnel. They teach your child the courses to prepare for the next grade, and you teach teachers about asthma so your child learns better. Too often, school personnel harbor outdated information and negative views about asthma. Or they panic at the thought of handling chronic disease. Rather than chance an attack, they keep your child from participating in activities.

Before the school year begins, request a meeting with the principal, classroom teacher, physical education teacher, and school nurse. Emphasize that you want to ease their job and help your child stay healthy. Reinforce that each student is unique, and you want to acquaint them with your child with asthma.

Bring general information about asthma (from your physician or asthma-related organization) that might help explain current thinking about this chronic disease. Stress that you have a normal youngster who can participate in most activities. Teachers just need to be alert to certain breathing difficulties that require quick and accurate assistance without panic. Your child's life depends upon their cooperation.

Be sure to mention symptoms that lead up to your child's attacks. Make special note of which signals require a call to parents and which demand emergency attention. Prepare a file of your child's medical information, lists of triggers, medications, and emergency telephone numbers. A copy should be kept in the school office, and one copy each in the classroom and gym.

Prepare a list of medications, schedules, and an inhaler to leave at school. Review your child's medications, what each does, and possible side effects. Mark each medication clearly with your child's name, teacher's name, and dosage. Demonstrate how your child should administer each one. Ask for cooperation in documenting any learning or behavior changes in reaction to medication changes.

Stress that your child must take medication at the first sign of asthma. Fill out any authorization forms necessary to permit your child to keep medication handy. Ensure that everyone understands that your child knows to stay calm, enlist an adult for help, and take medication independently.

Prepare a list of known asthma triggers. Identify items or foods your child should avoid. Ask if you could be notified of school construction or particular science projects that may introduce irritating substances into your child's environment. Explain that you would be happy to discuss alternate plans for your child's whereabouts, such as home study or working in another classroom, until the project is finished.

Plan for parties by preparing a packet of treats for your child that the teacher can store in class. When a surprise holiday or birthday party occurs, your child will not feel left out because he or she cannot eat some of the party items.

Decide whether exercise is an asthma trigger for your child. Discuss exercise-induced asthma symptoms with the physical education and regular education teacher. Emphasize that your child must have short-acting asthma medication handy during physical education classes, recess, or class outings.

Color-code your child's peak flow meter to indicate asthma severity zones and instructions. Explain what peak flow and the color coding mean. Show how the meter works. Tell school personnel that peak flow takes the guesswork out of asthma treatment, providing objective proof about the severity of your child's symptoms. Peak flow readings can aid in making decisions about participation in an activity school personnel may feel involves too much exertion.

If you expect that your child will have more than the usual amount of absences, discuss how your child can handle the missed work. Ask if you can pick up homework or if a work buddy could alert your child about homework or tests.

Misunderstandings are difficult for children with chronic disease. Classmates may:

- Tease your child about his or her lack of energy, asthma symptoms, and unusual inhalers
- Fear catching asthma
- Envy your child's missed school days or the extra attention an attack may bring
- Be jealous your child gets released from certain gym activities
- Reject your child because he or she is different

One way to ease asthma into the classroom is with humor and understanding. Ask the teacher if you and your child can explain asthma to the class. Have your child talk about what symptoms and episodes feel like. Have your child demonstrate measuring peak flow and inhaling medication.

Leave plenty of time for questions and answers. If your child has experienced unpleasant classmate interactions because of asthma, role-play some of these situations. Ask other students ways they would handle these situations. With younger classes, you may guide discussion more. But your older child may not want you within miles of the school.

Your Child's Asthma Away From Home

Older children can speak up for themselves. They know what triggers to avoid and they understand when to request an adult's assistance. They carry inhaler medication with them to prevent emergencies. But going to friends' homes may require advance planning for your preschooler or primary-grade child.

\ Call ahead. Alert other parents that your child has asthma and suggest that this is nothing to worry about. Explain your child's triggers and substances and situations to avoid. Tell the friend's parents where you will be in case of emergency. Let them know that should these precautions pose any problems, your child can stay home.

Make sure other parents know which food allergies your child has. Request that they do not tempt your child with foods that contain even the smallest amounts of these ingredients. Well-meaning people often think that a drop of an ingredient in an entire recipe could not possibly cause harm. But even the smallest bit of allergen can trigger strong reactions. Ask parents to contact you first if they have any doubts about foods or activities. Your child's health depends upon this cooperation.

Traveling With Allergic Youngsters

Traveling with children of any age can be complicated. Besides making vacation arrangements, you consider the interests of each family member. Now you need to plan for contingencies of asthma, too. Do not let an asthma attack mar your vacation. Remember to:

- Carry an extra supply of medications—one supply for luggage and one for handheld carry-on baggage. Bring along your emergency packet of information: insurance card and forms, physician's telephone number, and other pertinent information in your preventive treatment plan.

- Arrange to sit in nonsmoking sections of trains or overseas airplanes.
- Rent cars with air conditioning. Ask for cars used by non-smokers. If dealers assure you the smell will be gone, beware. They may use a strong cleaning solution that triggers worse symptoms than leftover smoke.
- Carry a supply of snack foods if your child has food allergies. Ask about ingredients that go into foods at restaurants and on airplanes. Packaged food bought on the road can be loaded with additives.
- Avoid vacations in places with high pollen counts or damp locations if your child has pollen or mold allergies.
- Prepare for visits to homes with pets or environments with vastly different vegetation. Talk with your physician about extra doses of preventive medication. Begin medication before you leave and continue after your return.
- Try to stay in newer and better-kept overnight accommodations. Older, cheaper hotels tend to have dusty, moldy heating systems and air conditioners. Be sure to request a nonsmoking room.
- Bring your child's nonallergenic pillow along. In fact, bring plenty of healthy diversions along so you all have a better time by keeping busy.

Common Asthma Myths

▶ *People who have asthma always wheeze.*

Wheezing is the high-pitched hissing sound someone makes when their airways are blocked. The strangled sound occurs as air rushes through narrowed passageways to and from the lungs. At one time, the medical community believed wheezing was asthma's trademark. Now physicians know that you can have asthma and not wheeze.

Wheezing results from several causes, only one of which is asthma. All these possibilities have something in common: blocked airways. Blockage with asthma can be anywhere in the airways—up in the voice box (larynx) or deep inside the bronchioles.

Whether or not someone wheezes has little bearing on where the blockage is or its severity. Sometimes airways are so blocked that no sound escapes. Similarly, airways can be extremely narrow yet not blocked enough to cause wheezing. Wheezing is actually a poor indicator of asthma and its severity.

▶ *People with asthma should refrain from exercise.*

In actuality, the reverse is true. Exercise is beneficial for everyone. Controlled exercise strengthens the heart and muscles and enhances overall well-being. For people with asthma, improved fitness reduces the risk of triggering an attack because people with asthma who are aerobically fit breathe easier during exercise, have fewer attacks, and need less medication.

Still, breathing needs to be monitored carefully during exercise and a treatment plan should be followed to prevent flare-ups. Asthma episodes from exercise are a sign that the disease is unstable and that treatments should be reviewed with a physician.

▶ *Only heavy exercise triggers exercise-induced asthma.*

Any activity can trigger asthma in someone who has exercise-induced asthma. Simple exertion, such as going upstairs or carrying groceries, can cause heavier breathing, which dries the airways. This prompts the airway muscles to tighten and mucous plugs to develop, similar to asthma induced by heavier exercise.

▶ *Asthma is all in your head.*

While the exact cause of asthma remains unclear, physicians know that asthma is a medical condition that affects pulmonary function. People with asthma have sensitive lungs that react to certain triggers and irritants. Airways tighten, swell, and fill with mucus, leading to trouble breathing and coughing or wheezing.

Still, strong emotions can affect breathing. The strain of yelling, crying, or laughing can stimulate nerves to cause muscle tightening, which could lead to asthma symptoms.

▶ *Parents cause asthma in their children.*

Asthma in children has always been a riddle. With so many unknowns, a likely source of blame for a child's condition has been the parents. Asthma can come from allergies, irritants, and exercise. These are concrete triggers that lead to real symptoms. Because asthma is a physical rather than psychological condition, parenting practices cannot bring about the disease.

▶ *People with asthma would be healthier moving to a different climate.*

Relocating seldom improves asthma. Some people find temporary relief from local pollen allergies. But allergy symptoms soon crop up with allergens in the new environment. A recent study surveyed 1,800 Scottish children who had moved. Researchers found that a new house exposed the children to different forms of pollutants, dust mites, and other allergens. There was a higher incidence of asthma, eczema, and other allergic conditions among children who lived in more than one home over a period of 12 to 14 years.

A person with asthma might find relief from cold air or big-city pollutants by moving. New forms of treatment, however, can reduce symptoms without uprooting a family.

▶ **Asthma attacks generally occur suddenly without warning.**

To onlookers, asthma appears to strike without warning. In reality, asthma gives several warning signs. These include a scratchy throat, fatigue, and chest tightness, and they precede more typical asthma symptoms of wheezing, coughing, and breathlessness. Someone with asthma will learn to recognize these signals and plan actions, such as medication or breathing exercises, to prevent a serious episode.

▶ **If you ignore your asthma symptoms, they will go away.**

Asthma is *not* a condition to ignore. Symptoms may only worsen with neglect, sometimes getting out of control. Asthma can become life-threatening. Attacks need immediate handling. Make sure a child with asthma knows to find medication and help from a parent, teacher, or friend at the first sign of illness.

9

◈

Common Questions and Answers About Asthma

Q. What is asthma?

A. Asthma is a chronic lung disease of the respiratory system that cannot be cured but can be controlled. Airways swell and narrow in response to certain triggers, making breathing difficult. Frequently, excess mucus and muscle tightening block the airways, further compromising airflow. These reactions result from airway sensitivity to a variety of irritants, such as exercise, cold air, pollens, and tobacco smoke.

Q. Is asthma hereditary?

A. Research indicates that in some people, asthma is hereditary. There is an increased likelihood of developing asthma if another family member has the disease. Scientists have discovered portions of genes, the message centers in each body cell, that cause allergy, which are forerunners of several asthma triggers. They identified other gene markers for asthma. Scientists believe that having both conditions doubles or triples the risk of asthma.

Additional evidence suggests that environment and social conditions play a role in developing breathing problems. Children who live in poorer or industrial neighborhoods are at greater risk of asthma. Scientists cannot say for sure why many asthma symptoms appear. But they continue to explore the mix of heredity and environment as strong indicators of respiratory diseases.

Q. Why do people get asthma?

A. Asthma indicates that the lungs are sensitive to inhaled substances known as triggers. Physicians are unclear about why some people get asthma and others do not. The reasons you have sensitive lungs vary with the type of asthma and symptoms you display. Your asthma could be the result of heredity, allergies, exercise, excessive exposure to irritants, or a combination of these factors. Any of these could trigger breathing problems in sensitive lungs. Nothing a person does or fails to do contributes to an asthma condition.

Q. Is asthma life-threatening?

A. Severe attacks that deprive the body of oxygen may be fatal. In 1996, almost 5,000 Americans died from asthma, and these numbers seem to be rising. Although death rates are low compared to the large numbers of people with asthma, these fatalities should not happen. Modern treatments are more effective than ever before, yet failure to control asthma accounts for most asthma deaths. If you take medication, monitor breathing, and seek help for worsening symptoms immediately, asthma will most likely not threaten your life.

Q. **Can people catch asthma?**

A. Asthma is not contagious. You cannot give people asthma by touching them or coughing into the air, as colds are transmitted. Similarly, you cannot catch asthma from someone else. Asthma is a condition that develops from inside someone's body.

Q. **Does asthma affect life span?**

A. Asthma that is under control should not have an impact on how long someone lives. Stable asthma prevents changes in the lungs and heart from low levels of oxygen. Older adults must take extra care, however, when asthma compounds other serious illnesses, such as heart disease and diabetes. Asthma adds to feelings of hopelessness and depression, which limits a person's overall ability to fight disease.

Q. **Will asthma go away?**

A. Unlike other lung diseases, asthma symptoms are reversible.

This means they come and go, depending upon exposure to certain triggers. Moreover, asthma symptoms tend to change, either improving or worsening over the years. Some children with asthma find their symptoms disappear, only to return in adulthood. The more severe the childhood asthma, the greater the likelihood of serious adult symptoms.

Q. How can someone control asthma?

A. The best way to control asthma is to follow the treatment plan devised with your physician. This involves identifying your asthma triggers and avoiding them whenever possible. It includes taking medication and learning to spot early signs of asthma so you can start treatment before symptoms worsen. The focus of treatment for stable asthma is prevention. Planning ahead for emergencies and being alert to increased symptoms show you are serious about controlling your asthma.

Q. Can a person with asthma still carry on regular activity?

A. The main goal of treatment is to control symptoms to lead a normal life. You can work, go to school, and exercise as long as you take precautions. Follow your medication plan, take flu shots, eat and sleep well, and exercise wisely. If you think you will encounter an asthma trigger, talk with your physician about an extra dose of medication. Plan ahead for unforeseen flare-ups, and they may not occur. By taking good care of yourself, you ensure that your days will be healthy and active.

Q. **Are asthma medications dangerous?**

A. Any medication is potentially dangerous. You and your physician will weigh the benefits of stabilizing your asthma with the risks of each medication. Certain medications, such as corticosteroids and theophylline, require constant monitoring because they can produce serious adverse effects. If you find your medication causes more problems than it solves, ask your physician to change it. Do not stop your medication until you have spoken with your doctor.

Q. **How can a child with asthma learn not to feel different?**

A. Every child is unique. Some wear glasses; others need braces; still others have freckles. If your child happens to have asthma, treat your child like any other growing girl or boy. Make sure your entire family understands the importance of following a treatment plan and keeping asthma symptoms under control. That way, your child can experience the joys and sorrows of growing up the same as any other child.

Resources

The organizations listed below can provide useful information, products, and services for people who have asthma. The books and videotapes listed can provide valuable information, support, and encouragement.

GENERAL HEALTH ORGANIZATIONS

These organizations provide free or reasonably priced print materials, videotapes, and educational programs on general aspects of asthma.

National Heart, Lung, and Blood Institute (NHLBI) Information
  Center
National Institutes of Health (NIH)
P.O. Box 30105
Bethesda, Maryland 20824-0105
phone: (301) 251-1222

WEB SITE:
  http://www.nhlbi.nih.gov/nhlbi/nhlbi.html

GOPHER SITE:
  gopher://fido.nhlbi.nih.gov:70/11/nhlbi

  Excellent national research resource and referral service; prepares helpful material, including booklets on starting an asthma support group and how to care for your child with asthma.

National Institute of Allergy and Infectious Diseases (NIAID)
Office of Communications
Building 31, Room 7A-50
31 Center Drive MSC
Bethesda, Maryland 20892-2520
phone: (301) 496-5717

E-MAIL:
ocpostoffice@flash.niaid.nih.gov

WEB SITE:
http://www.niaid.nih.gov

> Researches causes, prevention, and treatment of allergies; provides pamphlets for people with asthma and their families. Write for information and catalog.

Asthma and Allergy Foundation of America (AAFA)
1125 15th Street NW, suite 502
Washington, D.C. 20005
phone: (800) 7-ASTHMA or (202) 466-7643
fax: (202) 466-8940

E-MAIL:
info@aafa.org

WEB SITE:
http://www.aafa.org

> Produces bimonthly patient education newsletter filled with up-to-date asthma and allergy information; provides brochures and resource list of books and games that can be ordered at a discount to members.

American Lung Association (ALA)
1740 Broadway
New York, New York 10019-4374
phone: (800) 586-4872 or (212) 315-8700
fax: (212) 265-5642

WEB SITE:
http://www.lungusa.org

Call to locate the nearest affiliate.

National Jewish Medical and Research Center
1400 Jackson Street
Denver, Colorado 80206-2762
phone: (800) 222-5864 (Lung Line is a hot line for callers to hear the most recent facts about asthma) or (303) 388-4461

WEB SITE:
http://www.njc.org

Residential and outpatient treatment center; leader in asthma study and treatment.

American College of Allergy, Asthma and Immunology (ACAAI)
85 West Algonquin Road, suite 550
Arlington Heights, Illinois 60005
phone: (847) 427-1200
fax: (847) 427-1294

WEB SITE:
http://allergy.mcg.edu

Free asthma education kit and Life Quality (LQ) test, a 20-item questionnaire that can help people with asthma determine their fitness and recognize symptoms of poorly controlled asthma.

American Academy of Allergy, Asthma, and Immunology
611 East Wells Street
Milwaukee, Wisconsin 53202
phone: (800) 822-2762 or (414) 272-6071

WEB SITE:
http://www.aaaai.org

Provides information and referrals; has list of publications available for purchase.

Allergy and Asthma Network/Mothers of Asthmatics (AAN/MA)
3554 Chain Bridge Road, suite 200
Fairfax, Virginia 22030-2709
phone: (800) 878-4403 or (703) 385-4403
fax: (703) 352-4354

WEB SITE:
  http://www.podi.com/health/aanma

  Provides information, referrals, publication list of educational
  materials; sells peak flow meters; support organization.

ALTERNATIVE MEDICINE RESOURCES

American Academy of Medical Acupuncture
5820 Wilshire Boulevard, suite 500
Los Angeles, California 90036
phone: (800) 521-2262

WEB SITE:
  http://www.medicalacupuncture.org

  Telephone referral service for finding a local physician trained
  in acupuncture; limited resources for acupuncture education.

American Chiropractic Association
1701 Clarendon Boulevard
Arlington, Virginia 22209
phone: (703) 276-8800

WEB SITE:
  http://www.amerchiro.org

  Library includes materials on asthma and chiropractic and general information about chiropractors.

American Yoga Association
PO Box 19986
Sarasota, FL 34276
phone: (941) 953-5859

> Provides information; has list of publications available for purchase.

National Center for Homeopathy
801 North Fairfax Street, suite 306
Alexandria, Virginia 22314
phone: (703) 548-7790

E-MAIL:
nchinfo@igc.org

WEB SITE:
http://www.homeopathic.org

> Directory of homeopaths and general homeopathy information available for purchase.

WORKPLACE ORGANIZATIONS

A diagnosis of asthma can be tricky when triggers are job related. Once your asthma is under control, your next step is in adapting to the workplace. To do this, you need to know your rights. These organizations can provide the information you need to advocate on your own behalf.

Job Accommodation Network
918 Chestnut Ridge Road, suite 1
Morgantown, West Virginia 26506-6080
phone: (800) 526-7234 or (800) 526-2262 in Canada
Americans With Disabilities Act information: (800) 232-9675

E-MAIL:
jan@jan.icdi.wvu.edu

WEB SITE:

http://janweb.icdi.wvu.edu

International toll-free consulting service that provides information about job accommodations for employing people with disabilities and general employer/employee information.

Great Lakes Disability and Business Technical Assistance Center
Institute on Disability and Human Development (UAP)
College of Associated Health Professions
1640 Roosevelt Road (M/C 626)
Chicago, Illinois 60608
voice/teletypewriter (TTY): (800) 949-4232 or (312) 413-1407
fax: (312) 413-1856

WEB SITE:

http://www.gldbtac.org

Provides information on accommodating people with disabilities in the workplace.

US Equal Employment Opportunity Commission (EEOC)
1801 L Street NW
Washington, DC 20507
phone: (800) 669-6820
telecommunication device for the deaf (TDD): (800) 800-3302

WEB SITE:

http://www.eeoc.gov

Provides assistance in dealing with discrimination in the workplace.

YOUTH ORGANIZATIONS

Camps

Your child's asthma may be so severe that you worry about sending him or her away to camp. But there is no need to worry. There are more than

40 camps in the US specifically for children with respiratory problems. Staff members have the qualifications to handle your child's health requirements, and camp activities are organized around the needs of the children. To locate the camp nearest you, contact:

American Camping Association
5000 State Road 67 North
Martinsville, Indiana 46151
phone: (800) 428-2267

WEB SITE:

http://www.aca-camps.org

> The association checks each camp for such qualifications as safety standards. Then it publishes a yearly guide of accredited camps called *Guide to American Camping Association–Accredited Camps*. The guide contains more than 2,000 camps in the US. You can find the right camp for your child by looking in the index under "special clientele" and then locating "asthma—respiratory problems."

Advocacy and Education Programs

Kids on the Block
9385 C Gerwig Lane
Columbia, Maryland 21046
phone: (800) 368-KIDS (5437)

WEB SITE:

http://www.kotb.com

> Offers books, puppets, and videotapes about children with disabilities, including asthma; various local puppet troupes perform around the country.

ADULT BOOKS ON ASTHMA

Adams, Francis, MD. *The Asthma Sourcebook*. Chicago: Contemporary Books, 1995. Helpful information; thorough coverage.

Brookes, Tim. *Catching My Breath*. New York: Times Books, 1994. Tongue-in-cheek review of asthma information from someone with severe asthma who has been through many medical, scientific, and alternative medicine treatments; written by a journalist rather than a physician.

Friedewald, Vincent, MD. *Asthma*. Kansas City, MO: Andrews and McMeel, 1995. Multilist format for asthma overview.

Hannaway, Paul, MD. *The Asthma Self-Help Book*. Marblehead, MA: Lighthouse Press, 1989. Good overview; informative.

Harrington, Geri. *The Asthma Self-Care Book: How to Take Control of Your Asthma*. New York: HarperCollins, 1991. A self-help guide for people who have asthma.

Hogshead, Nancy, and Couzens, Gerald. *Asthma and Exercise*. New York: Henry Holt, 1990. An Olympic swimmer and writer explain asthma and how even athletes can overcome the effects of asthma and lead active lives.

Plaut, Thomas, MD. *Children With Asthma: A Manual for Parents*. Amherst, MA: Pedipress, Inc, 1988. Valuable information for parents of children with asthma; written from a doctor's perspective.

Plaut, Thomas, MD. *One-Minute Asthma*. Amherst, MA: Pedipress, Inc, 1995. A compilation of information on asthma.

Sander, Nancy. *A Parent's Guide to Asthma*. New York: Doubleday, 1988. Practical guide to parenting children with asthma from the founder of Mothers of Asthmatics (now Asthma and Allergy Network [AAN]).

Weinstein, Allan, MD. *Asthma*. New York: McGraw-Hill Publishing, 1987. One of the easiest to understand books for basic information on asthma. (Please consult other sources for information on the latest research and current medications.)

ALLERGY AND ALTERNATIVE
HEALING BOOKS

Allergy Information Association. *Food Allergy Cookbook: Diets Unlimited for Limited Diets.* New York: St. Martin's Press, 1983. Recommended food options for people with food allergies.

Astor, Stephen, MD. *Hidden Food Allergies.* Wayne, NJ: Avery Publishing Group, 1988. Guide to understanding a family member with food allergies.

Jelks, Mary, MD. *Allergy Plants That Cause Sneezing and Wheezing.* Tampa, Florida: World-Wide Publications, 1986.

McLain, Gary, PhD. *The Natural Way of Healing Asthma and Allergies.* New York: Dell Publishing, 1995. This book offers a variety of alternative remedies for asthma and allergies.

Meizel, Jane. *Your Food Allergic Child: A Parent's Guide.* Bedford, MA: Mill and Sanderson Publishing, 1990. Food preparation tips for planning safe meals for people with food allergies.

Scott, Julian. *Natural Medicine for Children* New York: William Morrow, 1990. Drug-free health care for children from birth to 12 years; homeopathy, massage, and other alternative remedies.

Tierra, Michael. *The Way of Herbs,* revised edition. New York: Pocket Books, 1990. Good general introduction to herbal healing.

Walsh, William. *The Food Allergy Book: Foods That Cause You Pain and Discomfort and How to Take Them From Your Diet.* St. Paul, MN: ACA Publications, 1995.

Weil, Andrew, MD. *Natural Health, Natural Medicine.* Sandy, OR: Eclectic Medical Publications, 1996. Good general introduction to the wellness perspective of alternative medicine.

ASTHMA BOOKS FOR YOUNG CHILDREN AND TEENS

Bergman, Thomas. *Determined to Win: Children Living With Allergy and Asthma.* Milwaukee, WI: Gareth Stevens, 1994 (primary grades).

Keller, Holly. *Furry.* New York: Greenwillow Books, 1992 (preschoolers; primary grades). A young girl's allergies make it difficult for her to find a pet.

Kerby, Mona. *Asthma.* New York: Franklin Watts, 1989 (junior high; high school). Overview of different types of asthma and their causes and treatments.

London, Jonathon. *The Lion Who Had Asthma.* Morton Grove, IL: Albert Whitman, 1992 (preschoolers).

Ostrow, William, and Ostrow, Vivian. *All About Asthma.* Morton Grove, IL: Albert Whitman, 1989 (grades 2 to 5). Written by a boy and his mother, complete with address where children can write to correspond with another child who has asthma; thorough coverage; easy to follow.

Rogers, Alison. *Luke Has Asthma, Too.* Burlington, VT: Waterfront Books, 1987. Reassuring story about two boys who have asthma.

Sanders, Nancy. *So You Have Asthma Too!* Fairfax, VA: Mothers of Asthmatics, 1988 (preschoolers; primary grades). Picture book about growing up with asthma.

Silverstein, Alvin and Virginia. *Asthma.* Springfield, NJ: Enslow Publishers, 1997 (middle grades).

Simpson, Carolyn. *Coping With Asthma.* New York: Rosen Publishing Company, 1995 (junior high; high school). General reference book.

Weiss, Jonathon. *Breathe Easy: Young People's Guide to Asthma.* New York: Magination Press, 1994.

VIDEOTAPES

Hogshead, Nancy with Drs. Stanley Wolf and Kathy Lampl. *Aerobics for Asthmatics*. From Aerobics for Asthmatics, Inc, 10301 Georgia Avenue, Suite 306, Silver Spring, Maryland 20902, (301) 681-6055. Forty-five-minute exercise tape by an Olympic gold medalist who has asthma; exercises help improve cardiovascular system and breathing.

Sanders, Nancy. *I'm a Meter Reader*. From Allergy and Asthma Network (AAN)/Mothers of Asthmatics, 3554 Chain Bridge Road, suite 200, Fairfax, Virginia 22030–2709, (800) 878-4403. Teaches children how to measure breathing with peak flow meters.

Glossary

This glossary defines terms that your doctor or your child's doctor may have mentioned or that you may have come across while reading about asthma. Italicized words within entries refer you to other entries for additional information.

A

acetylcholine: A chemical that transmits nerve impulses between cells.

active relaxation: Conscious tensing and relaxing of each muscle group to reduce stress.

acupuncture: An alternative medical treatment involving the insertion of special needles to treat illness and relieve pain.

adrenaline: A hormone produced by the adrenal glands; also called *epinephrine.*

aerosol inhalers: Widely used handheld devices that propel a mixture of medication in liquid propellant gas and preservatives into the lungs; *bronchodilators* and *anti-inflammatory* medications come in aerosol form.

airways: The network of passageways that transport air in and out of the *lungs* during breathing.

allergen: An invading substance that provokes an allergic reaction in some people.

allergist: A physician who specializes in the diagnosis and treatment of asthma and *allergies.*

allergy: Sensitivity to pollens, molds, foods, and other substances.

alveoli: Tiny air sacs deep inside the *lungs* where *oxygen* and *carbon dioxide* are exchanged during breathing.

antibody: A chemical in the *immune system* that binds to invading microorganisms and blocks their effects.

anticholinergics: A category of *bronchodilator* medications that help control muscle spasms.

antigen: An invading substance that causes the *immune system* to produce *antibodies* to fight it.

antihistamine: A medication that blocks the effects of the chemical histamine in the body, thereby reducing *allergy* symptoms.

anti-inflammatories: Drugs that reduce *airway* swelling.

atelectasis: Collapse of *lung* tissue caused by *airway* obstruction.

atopy: Another term for *allergy;* an increased tendency to form *antibodies* to common *allergens* that contribute to asthma.

B

barotrauma: Potentially fatal pressure injury caused by extreme changes in *lung* volume and outside air pressure, such as sometimes occurs in scuba diving.

beta$_2$ agonists: Drugs that stimulate certain sympathetic nerve-ending receptors (called beta$_2$ receptors) in the *lungs,* allowing the bronchial muscles to relax and the bronchial tubes to dilate.

brain: The control center of the *nervous system.*

bronchi: The branching system of *airways* in the *lungs.*

bronchial mucosa: The skinlike membrane that lines the *bronchi.*

bronchioles: The smallest *airways* in the pulmonary system.

bronchitis: Inflammation of the *trachea* and *bronchi.*

bronchoconstriction: Tightening of the *airways* in the *lungs.*

bronchodilators: Drugs that widen constricted *airways.*

bronchoscope: A thin tube that allows a physician to look inside the *lungs.*

bronchospasm: A muscle contraction that lessens airflow in the *lungs.*

butylated hydroxyanisole (BHA); butylated hydroxytoluene (BHT): Two chemicals added to grains and cereal products as preservatives that are known to cause allergic reactions in some people.

C

capillaries: Tiny blood vessels that connect the smallest veins and the smallest arteries.

carbon dioxide: A gas that is a byproduct of tissue metabolism; it is exhaled from the *lungs*.

cardiac asthma: Breathing problems caused by fluid buildup in the *lungs* as a result of *congestive heart failure*.

chemical challenge: A test in which a suspected or known asthma *trigger* is inhaled and then a pulmonary function test is given to measure the degree of sensitivity present.

cilia: Tiny, hairlike structures on the surface of certain cells; they move mucus through the respiratory tract with their wavelike motion.

congestive heart failure: A condition that occurs when the heart cannot pump enough blood to the *lungs* and the rest of the body, causing excess fluid to accumulate in the tissues.

corticosteroids: Drugs used to treat inflammation in asthma.

cross-reaction: Allergy symptoms resulting from foods in the same food family as a known *allergen*.

cyanosis: Bluish discoloration of the skin caused by low levels of *oxygen* in the blood.

cystic fibrosis: A genetic disease that causes excess mucus production in the respiratory tract, leading to persistent infections of the *lungs*.

cytokine: A chemical that kills or neutralizes substances invading the body.

D

decongestants: Drugs that reduce nasal congestion.

dypsnea: Difficulty breathing.

E

eczema: Skin inflammation.

electromyograph: Measurement of the electrical activity in muscle.

electrostatic precipitator: An air filter attached to a central heating unit that uses electric current to remove *allergens* from the air.

elimination diet: A diet used to determine food allergies and sensitivities; all suspected and possible food *triggers* are eliminated from the diet and reintroduced one at a time.

emphysema: A disease of the *alveoli* that results in shortness of breath.

endorphins: A natural substance produced in the brain that influences mood and perception of pain.

eosinophil: A type of white blood cell that increases in number during an allergic reaction.

eosinophil count: A test to measure the number of *eosinophils* in the bloodstream.

epinephrine: A hormone produced by the adrenal glands; also called *adrenaline.*

exercise challenge: A test involving physical exertion followed by a pulmonary function test to determine the presence of exercise-induced asthma.

exercise-induced asthma: Breathing problems caused by exercise.

expectorant: A medication that helps you cough up mucus.

extrinsic asthma: Asthma caused by *allergens* in the environment.

F

forced expiratory volume (FEV): The amount of air forced from the *lung* in 1 second.

forced vital capacity (FVC): Measurement of how long and how fully air can be blown out of the *lungs.*

formaldehyde: A gas that irritates the *airways;* it is given off by such things as building materials, home furnishings, permanent-press clothing, and cigarettes.

G

gene: The basic unit of heredity; each gene helps determine various inherited characteristics.

H

hay fever: Allergic reaction to airborne ragweed and other pollens; symptoms include runny nose, sneezing, and itchy, watery eyes.

heartburn: A burning sensation in the chest caused by a backup of stomach acid into the esophagus.

high-efficiency particulate air (HEPA) purifier: A special filter for vacuum cleaners, ventilation systems, and room air purifiers that traps air particles that are potential *allergens*.

homeopathy: A system of medicine in which extremely diluted solutions of natural substances ("remedies") are given to stimulate the person's "vital force."

hygrometer: An instrument that measures the amount of moisture in the air.

hyperreactivity: Sensitivity to an *allergen* that results in muscle contractions; in asthma, muscles tighten around the *bronchi*.

hyperventilation: Abnormal prolonged, rapid, and deep breathing.

hypocapnia: A shortage of *carbon dioxide* in the bloodstream due to impaired exchange of blood gases in the *alveoli* inside the *lungs*.

hypoxemia: A shortage of *oxygen* in the bloodstream due to impaired exchange of blood gases in the *alveoli* inside the *lungs*.

hypoxia: reduced levels of *oxygen* in body tissues.

I

immune system: A network of organs, cells, and glands that protect the body from infection.

immunoglobulin: Any of five different *antibodies* that block the effects of *antigens* in the body.

immunotherapy: Preventive therapy to desensitize a person's *immune system* to a known *allergen*.

inhaler: A medication delivery device that allows medicine to be breathed directly into the *lungs*.

intradermal test: An allergy skin test in which potential *allergens* are injected under the person's skin.

intrinsic asthma: Asthma caused by another disease or condition.

L

larynx: The voice box.

leukotrienes: A group of chemicals released from *mast cells* that cause harmful inflammation of the *bronchi* in asthma.

lungs: The two organs in the chest that take *oxygen* from the air and remove *carbon dioxide* from the body.

lymphocytes: White blood cells that are an essential part of the *immune system*.

M

mast cells: A type of cell that secretes substances that can cause redness and swelling during an allergic reaction.

mediators: Substances released by *mast cells* when stimulated that can cause redness and swelling during an allergic reaction.

meditation: A state of relaxation brought about by concentration on an object, word, or phrase.

methylxanthines: *Bronchodilator* drugs that relax *airway* muscles to increase airflow.

mildew: A form of fungus that grows indoors under moist conditions.

monosodium glutamate (MSG): A food additive that can cause asthma, headache, diarrhea, nausea, sweating, and skin irritation.

mucous glands: Glands embedded in the bronchial lining that keep *airways* lubricated with mucus so that harmful substances can be easily eliminated from the *lungs*.

N

nasal polyps: Small fleshy growths inside the nose that may develop as a result of continuous inflammation of the mucous membrane.

nebulizer: A device used to administer *aerosol bronchodilator* drugs through a face mask; it is used especially for emergency treatment of severe asthma.

nervous system: The body's control center, composed of the brain, *spinal cord,* and nerves.

neurotransmitters: Chemicals that carry messages between nerve cells or from nerve cells to other cells.

nitrogen dioxide: A gas emitted from gas appliances (for example, a kitchen stove) that can impair breathing.

O

occupational asthma: Asthma caused by exposure to *allergens* in the workplace.

otitis media: Middle ear inflammation caused by an upper respiratory tract infection.

otolaryngology: The medical specialty that deals with allergic, inflammatory, and other diseases of the ears, nose, and throat (ENT).

oxygen: An essential gas that enters the bloodstream through the *lungs* to nourish body tissues.

P

parabens: A group of preservatives found in food and medications that may cause swelling, redness, and painful skin irritation in some people.

parasympathetic nervous system: The part of the *nervous system* that tightens the bronchial tubes and decreases blood pressure and heart rate.

particulates: Fine particles in the air that are produced by fuel combustion and contribute to air pollution.

passive relaxation: A relaxation technique in which the mind focuses on a phrase or sound and contributes to muscle relaxation and easier breathing.

peak flow meter: A device used to measure the rate at which a person can exhale.

pharynx: The throat.

pneumonia: Inflammation of the *lungs,* usually caused by an infection.

postural drainage: A technique for dislodging mucus from the *lungs* by positioning the body so that drainage can occur.

prick test: An allergy skin test in which an *allergen* is placed on the skin and the skin is pierced lightly with a needle; the person is then monitored for a possible allergic reaction.

pulmonary disease: Diseases and conditions that affect the *lungs,* such as asthma, emphysema, and chronic *bronchitis.*

pulmonologist: Doctor who specializes in diseases and disorders of the *lungs.*

pulse oximetry: A testing device that clips onto an earlobe or fingertip to measure *oxygen* levels in the blood.

R

radioallergosorbent test (RAST): A laboratory test used to identify allergy to specific substances by measuring immunoglobulin E (IgE, a protein found in white blood cells) levels in the blood.

reflux: Backward flow, as in reflux esophagitis, which is the backward flow of stomach acid into the esophagus.

respirator: A machine that pumps air in and out of the *lungs* of a person who has lost the ability to breathe.

respiratory system: The body system that carries *oxygen* from the air to the bloodstream and removes the waste product *carbon dioxide*.

rhinitis: Allergic inflammation of the mucous membrane that lines the nose.

S

scratch test: An allergy skin test in which the skin is scraped and a specific *allergen* is dropped onto the scraped area and then monitored for a possible reaction.

spacer: A device that attaches to an *inhaler* to direct medication into the *lungs;* it limits medication lost in the mouth and the amount of mouth bacteria entering the *lungs*.

spinal cord: The nerve tissue that runs down the central canal in the spine and transmits messages from the brain to the rest of the body.

spirometer: An instrument used to measure the amount and speed of air inhaled and exhaled from the *lungs*.

spirometry: Tests of *lung* air capacity and pulmonary function performed with a *spirometer*.

status asthmaticus: A life-threatening, prolonged asthma attack; this is a medical emergency.

steroids: See *corticosteroids*.

strep throat: A bacterial infection of the throat.

stridor: Noisy breathing, often caused by obstruction or inflammation of the *larynx*.

sulfites: A group of preservatives added to foods and medications that can trigger allergic asthma in some people.

sweat test: A test for *cystic fibrosis* that measures salt content in sweat.

sympathetic nervous system: The part of the *nervous system* that raises blood pressure and heart rate and widens the bronchial tubes.

syndrome: Signs and symptoms occurring together that indicate a specific disease.

T

t'ai chi: Chinese martial arts system of coordinated movements; may help reduce stress and expand *airways*.

tartrazine (FD & C yellow dye #5): Food coloring known to cause an allergic asthma reaction in some people.

thrush: A common yeast infection of the mouth and back of the throat; also called candidiasis.

trachea: The large *airway* that connects the *larynx* to the *bronchi*; also called the windpipe.

triggers: Irritants to the *lungs* that cause symptoms of asthma.

U

upper airways: Passageways into and out of the *lungs,* including the nose, mouth, and throat.

W

wheals: Raised, itchy, red patches of skin that sometimes have a pale center; they are sometimes triggered by allergic reactions; also called hives.

Y

yoga: Hindu philosophy system involving meditation exercises that combine deep breathing and muscle strength and flexibility exercises; may help increase airflow and reduce stress.

Index